PREDICTING
READING FAILURE

PREDICTING READING FAILURE

A Preliminary Study

•

by

KATRINA DE HIRSCH

JEANNETTE JEFFERSON JANSKY

and

WILLIAM S. LANGFORD

•

A HARPER INTERNATIONAL EDITION

jointly published by

Harper & Row, *New York, Evanston & London*

and John Weatherhill, Inc., *Tokyo*

In GRATITUDE TO A.R.

The research reported herein was performed pursuant to Contract U-1270, Health Research Council of the City of New York.

This Harper International Edition is an unabridged, photo-offset reproduction of the American edition. It is for sale in Japan by JOHN WEATHER-HILL, INC., *50 Ryudo-cho, Azabu, Minato-ku, Tokyo; in the United Kingdom and on the continent of Europe by* HARPER & ROW, LTD., *69 Great Russell Street, London W.C. 1; and in other designated countries by* HARPER & ROW, PUBLISHERS, INCORPORATED, *49 East 33rd Street, New York, N.Y. 10016 /* *Library of Congress catalog card number 66-22045 / Printed in Japan / First printing, April, 1967.*

Contents

•

Foreword

◆

The basic concepts implicit in this study emerge as important contributions to the field of language disorders. The study shows that children mature physiologically and psychologically along foreseeable lines and that those children who lag severely in over-all maturation can be predicted to fail academically. At the heart of the authors' contribution is the demonstration that valid predictions of reading, spelling, and writing achievement can be made by evaluating children's perceptual, motor, and language behavior at early ages.

While the authors have used modern research and statistical tools in developing their findings, they have supplemented these methods with clinical observations of the children studied, drawing upon their many years of clinical experience with every variety of language disturbance. Thus the book provides an imaginative and insightful picture of the children, based on the authors' personal relationships with them over a period of two and one-half years.

A specific contribution is the construction of a predictive index consisting of a simple battery of tests for use by schools. This index, which is now being validated, is designed to enable teachers to identify, before the beginning of first grade, those children who present a high risk of academic failure.

And there is a bonus. The authors have studied a group of prematurely born children and compared their learning patterns with those of children born at term. Their findings in this area throw light on the significance of the kind of maturational delays found in many prematurely born children and the relationship of these delays to learning.

Maturation is determined by a variety of factors: inherited patterns, biological growth, and the child's specific life experiences—emotional, cultural, and educational. The rate of maturation varies from child to child, and education, if it is to be effective, must take such variations into account. Special educational techniques are essential for children who suffer from maturational lags. The authors describe a number of such techniques which should be helpful in preparing these children better for learning and thus preparing them better for living.

DR. LAURETTA BENDER

June 1966

Acknowledgments

—

This research was made possible by the generous support of the Health Research Council of the City of New York. Grateful acknowledgment is due, too, to the Aaron Norman Foundation, which, through the good offices of Frank A. Weil, provided the initial funds that enabled us to get started. The assistance of Mrs. Augusta Lyons and of the late Mrs. Hopkins Ford is greatly appreciated.

The warm interest and constant encouragement of Drs. Edward Curnen, Rustin McIntosh, Richard Masland, Houston Merritt, Sidney Carter, William Silverman, George Mirick, Alfred Freedman, and George Carden have sustained us over many ups and downs during the past three years.

This study would not have been possible without the contribution of two dedicated research assistants, Natalie Garik, M.A., and Jeane Gazdag, M.A. They carried out much of the testing of the children, and the fact that there was so little attrition in the group is largely due to their clinical skill. Mrs. Garik, in addition, analyzed all tape recordings of the children's stories and labored in the library. Mrs. Gazdag visited over one hundred schools and collected much important information from the teachers.

We owe thanks to Dr. Cynthia Deutsch for advice in the

initial stages of the study, and to Dr. Helen Schucman for her able assistance during the first year. Our thanks, above all, are due to E. David Nasatir, who acted as our statistical consultant. The statistical aspects of the study owe everything to his incisiveness, as well as to his ingenuity, patience, and devotion. Any flaws in the presentation of the data are entirely ours.

Mrs. Theodore Pockman's editorial help was invaluable.

Dr. Dorothea McCarthy's gracious readiness to answer questions was greatly appreciated.

We owe thanks to Mrs. Marian Carr, Mrs. Frederick Hurd, and Mrs. John S. Dorf for their cheerful help in the academic testing of the children.

We are deeply grateful to three people who gave so generously of their time and provided constructive and much needed criticism: Dr. Hildred Schuell, Dr. Ruth Blunden, and Mrs. Richard Masland.

Our gratitude, finally, goes to the cooperative parents and to their lively and entertaining children.

Introduction

●

One of today's major social problems is the enormous number of children who, as a result of severe reading, writing, and spelling disabilities, are unable to realize their intellectual and educational potentials. The incidence of reading difficulties has been reported to be as high as 30 per cent of the school population (191, 197)[*]; more conservative estimates put the figure between 5 per cent and 15 per cent (100, 188). According to the National Council of Teachers of English (216) this would mean that at least 4 million elementary school children in the United States are disabled readers. "The magnitude of the reading problem and the shattering impact of reading disability on personal and vocational adjustment should accord proposals for its correction a major position in mental hygiene programs," states Leon Eisenberg (63), professor of child psychiatry at Johns Hopkins, in highlighting the urgency of the problem.

This book is concerned with young children's failure to master reading, writing, and spelling. Failure to cope with printed and written language, can, however, be understood only if viewed as one aspect of a more comprehensive disturbance.

[*] Numbers in parentheses refer to the corresponding works listed in References Cited.

Spoken language precedes written and printed forms of verbal symbolic behavior. In the short span between eighteen and forty months the child weaves an enormous number of phonemic symbols into the pattern of spoken language—a formidable task and one fraught with hazards.

Children seen in clinical practice may show a variety of verbal-symbolic disturbances (177). There are some with adequate intelligence and essentially intact hearing who at the expected age or much later fail partially or entirely to interpret or use the language of their culture. They fail not because of physical disabilities—such failures belong in a different category—but because they have difficulties with the decoding and encoding of verbal symbols; they do not pay attention to information fed through auditory pathways; they hear, but they do not necessarily understand (121). Their intake is diffuse and undifferentiated. To them both the configuration of the word and its meaning are highly unstable, and this instability seems to be related to their inability to assign consistent symbolic significance to input events. These children's verbal output reflects their diffuse reception. Speech may be replaced by jargon; it may be drastically limited in quantity and crude and undifferentiated in quality. Most of these youngsters eventually learn to use verbal tools. However, limited verbalization, grammatical defects, and often crippling deficits in the printed and written forms of language usually follow in the wake of prolonged delay in language comprehension and use.

There is another group of children who by and large understand spoken language and who do talk, but who, long after the age of four, are still more or less unintelligible. Many have a history of delayed speech development. Their verbalizations are replete with distortions, omissions, and substitutions of sounds and are only primitive and crude approximations of the correct model. Their failure to grasp essential syntactical concepts, furthermore, testifies to their inability to master the linguistic code. Such children's difficulties recede with maturation. However, articulatory immaturities and trouble with the formulation and organization of both spoken and written language are observable at later ages.

One finds similar deficits in the organization of spoken and written language in a third group—the so-called cluttering children (241). Their speech is characterized by fluctuations in rate, by rhythmic disorders, and by a tendency to scramble the order of sounds, syllables, and words. Most clutterers present spelling disabilities, and their jerky, dysrhythmic handwriting mirrors their disorganized speech.

Underlying such disturbances in spoken language are deviations in perceptuomotor and behavioral organization. Among language-handicapped children one encounters many who are hyperactive and explosive and who find it difficult to channel impulses and integrate behavior. These children's central nervous system patterning seems to be immature. They show difficulties with fine motor control, a crude body image, and primitive visuomotor experiences, all testifying to the fact that severe deficits in oral language are part of a generalized developmental dysfunction.

The essential feature in verbal behavior, according to Richard Masland (162), is the sequencing of auditory events. Children suffering from disorders of spoken language distort the sequence of auditory verbal signals. The short auditory memory span and the tendency to scramble words and sounds, which is so characteristic a feature in speech-defective youngsters, point to basic difficulties in *temporal organization.*

The overwhelming majority of children suffering from *spoken* language disorders often present difficulties also with the decoding and encoding of *printed and written* language—with reading, writing, and spelling. Poor readers have, of course, trouble primarily with the processing of information received through *visual* pathways, and disturbances in *spatial* organization are in the foreground. However, as Karl Lashley (146) points out, temporal and spatial order are nearly interchangeable, and in learning to read, the young child has to translate a sequence of sounds seen—a sequence in space—into a sequence of sounds heard—a sequence in time.

Spoken, printed, and written language difficulties all involve disturbances of sequential behavior (177); such disturbances tend to be pervasive and seem to reflect subtle deviations in the developmental process. As does Lauretta Bender (12), we look on reading, writing, and spelling difficulties as belonging to the broader category of *developmental* disturbances.

Because emotional problems are frequent concomitants of severe language disorders, it has been assumed that *all* difficulties in verbal-symbolic functioning are psychologically determined. While it is true that lack of communicative drive and affective disturbances are at the root of *some* language and learning dysfunctions, psychological problems may *result* from massive difficulties with the comprehension and use of verbal symbols. The inability of speech-deprived children to discharge tension and anxiety by way of words and to verbalize anger and aggression may force them to resort to action and may keep them tied to developmentally more archaic forms of coping. Lack of serviceable communicative tools hampers developing ego functions of mastery, impulse control, and ability to postpone gratification.

Children with reading disabilities are not as totally disabled emotionally as are youngsters who lack words for expression and communication. Nevertheless, reading failure frequently results in an impaired self-image, and many children become social and emotional casualties as a result of early defeat (97). Arthur Gates (75) notes that 75 per cent of the youngsters with "specific" reading disturbances develop marked signs of maladjustment. In her study of the personality patterns of children with severe reading difficulties, Gladys Natchez (170) speaks of their intense anxiety and concludes that concerted efforts will have to be directed toward prevention.

Adverse emotional reactions to reading failure appear very early in the elementary grades and complicate primary difficulties with verbal symbolic functioning. It is therefore essential to identify children destined to fail at the earliest possible moment. In Sweden prompt identification and remediation has led to a drastic reduction of reading disabilities (159). Preventive steps are being taken in Belgium (163) and have been strongly recommended by Borel-Maisonny (26) and a group of educational psychologists in France (212).

Ralph Rabinovitch and his associates (189) have stated that it is essential to develop diagnostic criteria of future failure at early ages. This book represents an attempt to establish such criteria and to determine whether a distinct and identifiable pattern of perceptuomotor and oral language deficits at preschool age is *predictive* of difficulties with visual language—with reading, writing, and spelling—in subsequent years.* Such criteria would enable educators to identify at kindergarten level, "high-risk" children—that is to say, those in danger of failing when they are exposed to formal education.

* It is emphasized here that this study is *preliminary* in nature; the results are now being validated on 400 children in New York City.

PREDICTING
READING FAILURE

1
Background and Rationale

A growing number of schools (6) assess children's readiness for formal education by one of three procedures: reading readiness tests, intelligence evaluations (usually of a group variety), and informal evaluation of the child by the kindergarten teacher. While all three of these measures have proved their usefulness, each has certain limitations.

Existing reading tests, according to Jeanne Chall and Florence Roswell (39), do not lend themselves easily to the formulation of specific educational strategies. Most tests, moreover, do not predict performance in the areas of writing and spelling.

On the other hand, the use of intelligence tests for prediction has been challenged (94) on the ground that reading difficulties occur among children at virtually all intellectual levels. An intelligence quotient, furthermore, represents a global rather than a differentiated evaluation of a child's potential and fails to take into account some aspects of perceptual functioning that seem to be important determinants in early reading success or failure.

Finally, the individual kindergarten teacher's assessment of the child, although often remarkably accurate (6, 104, 136), represents an essentially subjective judgment, one that cannot readily be duplicated. Moreover, not all teachers possess the training, intuition, or experience that would enable them to make a reliable evaluation of a child's readiness.

A number of researchers have attempted clinical (37, 111) and statistical predictions of reading performance. (A predictive investigation, as defined by Alexander Thomas, Herbert Birch, and their collaborators (229), utilizes a set of analyzed initial findings to anticipate the nature of an eventual state.) Some have used single variables—such as auditory discrimination (230), visuomotor competence (143), the anxiety level of the child (42), or his self concept (238) as demonstrated in kindergarten or early first grade—to predict reading performance nine to twelve months later. Clyde Martin (160) and other researchers (184, 211) have relied on batteries of predictive tests. One of the earliest and best instruments is Marian Monroe's (166).* During the course of our investigation several test batteries predicting reading performance have appeared; the most inclusive, by Max Weiner and Shirley Feldmann (240), consists of eight perceptual and language tasks; another, by Thomas Barret (8), uses a variety of visual discrimination tests, and there is now an instrument being developed by Chall and her associates (39).

This investigation differs from others of its kind in three important respects: It explores a larger sector of the child's perceptuomotor and oral-language organization than do other studies; it predicts spelling and writing achievement in addition to reading; and, finally, the interval between prediction and outcome is more than twice as long as in most other studies.

This study evolved out of our experience with children at the Pediatric Language Disorder Clinic, Babies Hospital, Columbia-Presbyterian Medical Center, New York. We worked with groups of intelligent four- and five-year-old youngsters who had been referred initially because of oral-language deficits. An extraordinarily large proportion of the children developed reading, writing, and spelling difficulties several years later.

---

* Anna Gillingham's unpublished predictive battery was put into use by the Sidwell-Friends School in Washington, D.C., the Francis Parker School in Chicago, and a public school system in Seattle.

The clinical impression of these youngsters was one of striking immaturity. Their performance resembled that of chronologically younger subjects not only in oral language, but also in a variety of perceptuomotor tasks. So frequently was this pattern encountered that it raised the question of whether neurophysiological immaturity, as reflected in relatively primitive perceptuomotor and oral-language functioning, might be linked to subsequent deficits in reading, writing, and spelling, all of which require a high degree of differentiation and integration.

We recognize that a variety of social (55), environmental (133), and psychological (22, 152) factors are significant in the acquisition of reading skills, and we concur with Abraham Fabian (65), who maintains that learning to read requires the developmental timing and integration of both neurophysiological and psychological aspects of readiness. Nevertheless, we limited ourselves to the preschool child's perceptuomotor and linguistic functioning, because in this area we had found considerable deviation from the norm among children who subsequently failed in reading and spelling. We therefore put together a battery of tests which we hoped would reflect the children's perceptuomotor and linguistic status at kindergarten level. Performance on these tests, combined with clinical evaluation of the children, did, in fact, prove to be effective in predicting reading and spelling difficulties in the group originally referred because of oral-language deficits.

However, results led to a series of new questions: Would the tests by themselves, unsupported by experienced clinical judgment, be equally effective for prediction? Would the tests predict successfully for a *general* as opposed to a clinical population? Would certain tests predict more reliably than others? And finally, would such tests in combination yield a predictive instrument of widespread applicability?

The principle aims of the study, then, were threefold:

To determine to what extent certain tests administered at kindergarten age to a sample from the general population predict reading, writing, and spelling achievement two and a half years later, at the end of the second grade;

To single out from these tests those most effective for prediction;

To combine the best predictors into an instrument that could be used for the identification of "high-risk" children.

To determine the predictive efficacy of the kindergarten tests for a *clinical* population was an additional aim of the investigation. In the search for such a clinical group, it seemed desirable to choose a sample different from the speech-defective one originally studied. A group of prematurely born children was available at the Babies Hospital for research. In view of our theoretical bias, these prematurely born children were of particular interest, because they are assumed to start life with neurophysiological lags and are reported to show more reading disabilities than can be expected in a general sample. A group of prematurely born children, then, was selected to represent a clinical population.

2
Selection Procedures and Tests

◆

SELECTION OF CHILDREN

Children who had been born between September 1, 1955, and June 30, 1956, who weighed over 2,500 grams (5 pounds, 8 ounces) at birth, and who had participated in the Fetal Life Study carried out between 1953 and 1955 at Babies Hospital, Columbia-Presbyterian Medical Center, New York City, were placed in a selection pool. (The children in this population had originally been chosen at random from admissions to the Sloane Antepartum Clinic.) From this pool were drawn those children who: (1) came from homes in which English was the predominant language spoken; (2) rated IQs within one standard deviation above and below 100 (IQs of 84 to 116), as obtained on Form L of the Stanford-Binet Intelligence Scale (1937 revision); (3) presented no significant sensory deficits; and (4) showed no evidence of psychopathology, as judged clinically.

Considerable evidence testifies to the fact that a foreign-language background is a handicap when it comes to mastering skills such as reading, writing, and spelling (34, 155) that are largely culturally determined. Thus, Puerto Rican youngsters who are chiefly exposed to Spanish are clearly at a disadvantage when they encounter printed or written English. Their reading performance cannot, in all fairness, be compared with that of their peers who use English as their main tool for communication.

Sensory deficit was another reason for excluding some children. Macdonald Critchley (47) has discussed the significance for reading of visual defects. A number of investigators (41, 194) have found farsightedness, lack of binocular vision, eye-muscle imbalance, or slow fusion to be associated with reading disorders. Others (44, 83, 84, 173, 231) have taken the position that mild visual deficits, variations in eye movements, or eye-muscle imbalance do not necessarily interfere with reading, which is essentially a perceptual function involving central processes. That faulty eye movements are the *result* rather than the *cause* of poor reading is the position of some researchers (225, 235). The 1940 report of the Ophthalmological Section of the Los Angeles County Medical Association states: ". . . If the visual acuity is reduced 50% or more, the child will have difficulty in interpreting symbols because he cannot see well. . . . Except in far-sightedness and astigmatism of a marked degree, the child's power of focusing is sufficient to give adequate though not perfect vision, and a small amount of myopia may even be an advantage rather than a disadvantage in reading. The presence of a crossed eye with normal vision in one eye has little or no effect on reading ability. . . . Compensated muscle imbalance, such as phorias of a marked degree, does not affect interpretation of symbols. . . . So-called 'faulty' eye movements, as judged by regressions, depend primarily on poor visual understanding of subject matter read and not on incoordinated eye muscles. . . . Not the eyes, but the brain learns to read." (See Rodman Irvine, "An Ocular Policy for Public Schools," *American Journal of Ophthalmology*, 24 (1941), 779–788.)

We share Donald Leton's (150) and Frances Ilg's and Louise Ames's (118) position that certain deficiencies in oculomotor skills are related to delayed maturation of neuromuscular function rather than to peripheral visual defects. Visual functions are still maturing between the ages of five and seven, and they were therefore subject to change during the period covered by the present study. Assessment of visual function was thus limited to a simple test of visual acuity, as measured by the American Optical Company Kindergarten Chart. Children whose acuity was less than 20/40, and those whose behavior during the testing session suggested visual disturbance, were referred for ophthalmological evaluation. If the ophthalmologist considered the child's vision to be inadequate for educational purposes, the child was removed from the sample.

Even a moderate hearing loss in young children can be assumed to interfere with reading and spelling. Those children, therefore, who showed deficits in auditory acuity on a whisper test, or those in whom clinical observation suggested lowered auditory thresholds, were referred for audiological investigation. Children whose hearing was judged to be inadequate for functioning in the classroom were excluded.

Children with intellectual endowment considerably above or below average were not included in the study. We excluded "high IQ" children because little is known about the way highly intelligent children compensate for initial perceptuomotor lags. "Slow" children were excluded because they could not have been expected to master reading skills at the age investigated here. Limiting the group to subjects with IQs one standard deviation above and below 100, moreover, resulted in a relatively homogeneous population in terms of intellectual endowment.

The role of psychopathology as a cause of reading difficulties has been discussed by many authors (22, 181). A distinction has been made in the literature between "specific" reading, writing, and spelling disorders, and learning disabilities that are related to ego impairment (40, 114, 188). Gerald Pearson (181) says that, in the latter, the dominance of "primary processes" interferes with the ability to utilize information (as they do, for instance, in the child for whom the printed letters on the page represent hostile and threatening forces). Since some learning difficulties can be assumed to reflect a general disturbance in ego development and ego functioning, children who clinically presented severe psychopathology were excluded from the study.

At the time of the kindergarten testing, the median age of the 53 children was 5 years, 10 months; two-thirds of the sample were concentrated in the relatively narrow range of 5 years, 8 months, to 6 years, 1 month. The youngest child was 5 years, 2 months, and the oldest was 6 years, 6 months old.

Thirty boys and 23 girls participated in the project. Negro children constituted 40 per cent of the sample; 85 per cent of the children attended kindergarten.

The educational attainments of the children's parents placed them predominantly in the lower middle class. Fifty-six per cent had completed high school but not college; 42 per cent had less than a high school education; only 2 per cent were college graduates. In comparison, among New York City adults in 1962, only 29 per cent had completed high school, but not college; 63 per cent had not finished high school; 8 per cent were college graduates (233). The group of parents in the study was thus relatively homogeneous, more of the individuals being in the middle group and fewer at either extreme. The group's lower middle class character is further borne out by the parents' occupations. Of the breadwinners (almost all fathers), 72 per cent were in lower middle class jobs: clerical and sales work, skilled trades, and operatives of moving machinery; another 15 per cent were small business proprietors or managers. In general, then, the children represented neither the culturally deprived nor the culturally privileged, but a fairly typical lower middle stratum of an urban society.

BACKGROUND INFORMATION

This research effort, like others of its kind, was dependent on the parents' willingness to bring in their children for testing, often at considerable inconvenience to themselves. Parents who are willing to participate in a longitudinal study of this kind are undoubtedly interested in their children's welfare and success, but they are probably also somewhat anxious and concerned over performance. We made an effort to dissipate anxiety when necessary, and to provide support without encouraging dependence.

A positive relationship between the staff and the parents and children was fostered by the private-office setting in which the testing took place. Most parents enjoyed the friendly and comfortable atmosphere provided for them, and the children were usually eager to come back to play with the toys. There was remarkably little attrition in the group: The only child to drop out of the general sample was a member of a family that moved away.

Certain kinds of background information were obtained from the parents and were included for correlation with later achievement because of the many reports which emphasize that there exists an association between such background factors and subsequent reading competence.

One of the factors is the *family history* of language and handedness. Samuel Orton (175) and researchers such as Bertil Hallgren (90) and Knud Hermann and Edith Norrie (106) have all stressed genetic aspects of reading disabilities. Arthur Drew (59) has suggested that the disturbance in Gestalt functioning, which he believed to play a crucial role in reading disorders, might be inherited as a dominant trait. In view of these considerations, information was obtained as to speech, reading, writing, and spelling difficulties of the parents, their siblings, and their children—as well as to ambidexterity or left-handedness in the immediate family.

Furthermore, data on certain aspects of *environmental stimulation* were collected for correlation with later achievement. One was the parents' educational attainment. Another was the child's ordinal position in the family, since some researchers (98, 179, 199) have found that younger children are generally poorer learners than their older siblings. Maternal employment was felt to be important—Dorothea McCarthy (156) postulates a gradient of verbal sufficiency that is dependent on the frequency and quality of the mother's contact with the child. Finally, exposure and response to stories (165) and television were recorded, as was kindergarten attendance (34, 54).

Other background variables explored in terms of their efficacy as predictors were *intelligence*, chronological *age*, and *sex*. Vance Hall (89) reported that almost three times as many boys as girls are held back in the elementary grades. Because the literature reports differences between Negro and Caucasian children in the area of oral language (36, 55), the two groups' performance on written and printed language tests was compared here.

TESTING

Testing involved four visits over a period of nearly three years. Each session lasted from one to two-and-a-half hours. The first interview was used to obtain background information, to assess the children in terms of vision, hearing, and intelligence, and to screen out possible psychopathology. During the second session, the large battery of kindergarten tests was administered. The children were, finally, re-evaluated once at the end of their first and once at the end of their second year of school.

THE KINDERGARTEN TESTS

The selection of the kindergarten tests reflects the authors' theoretical position, which is derived from Jean Piaget (185), Arnold Gesell (78), Heinz Werner (246), and Lev Vygotsky (236), who postulate evolving stages in sensorimotor, perceptual, and linguistic functioning. We assumed that a child's perceptuo-motor and language level at kindergarten age forecasts his later performance on such highly integrated tasks as reading, writing, and spelling. In order to assess this level, a wide range of tests of varying complexity was administered. Although some were expected to be less predictive than others, the choice was based on the belief that each reflected, in some measure, the child's perceptuomotor and linguistic competence.

The thirty-seven kindergarten tests are described in the following pages. Many, but not all, are standardized or were adapted from standardized instruments; others were devised by the writers. A detailed description of scoring procedures for the ten tests chosen for the Predictive Index is included in Appendix II, and a description of the other twenty-seven is available.

Behavioral Patterning

TEST 1. *Hyperactivity, Distractibility, and Disinhibition*

When the child enters first grade he is expected to pattern his behavior in a way which will allow him to focus on the educational task ahead. While hyperactivity, distractibility, and disinhibition are normal features in very young children, a modicum of control is expected at kindergarten age. It was assumed that lack of such control at this level would augur poorly for subsequent academic performance. Observations of the children's behavior extended over the entire testing period.

Motility Patterning

TEST 2. *Concomitant Movements*

The number of concomitant movements was noted during balancing, drawing, tongue flection, and writing.

Teicher (226) discusses the progression of children's motility patterning, which approaches that of the adult in adolescence. Much of the toddler's behavior is global and involves activity of the total organism. Global motility presumably reflects immature central nervous system organization, and a number of researchers (12, 43) have observed a relationship between undifferentiated motility and reading disorders.

Gross Motor Patterning

TESTS 3, 4, *and* 5. *Balance, Hopping, and Throwing*

Two of N. Oseretzky's tests (178), Balance and Hopping, were selected for the investigation of gross motor coordination, and a Throwing test was added.

Gesell (79) maintains that postural skills ". . . serve as an essential preparation for the development of the . . . more refined skills of later years. Writing, for example, is a highly specialized activity which can be successfully undertaken only when certain earlier acquired skills such as . . . sitting balance are so well mechanized that they do not interfere with the writing activity." Since acquisition of certain gross motor skills thus seemed to be a prerequisite for academic functioning, tests of gross motor performance were included in the battery.

Fine Motor Patterning

For investigation of fine motor skills, the children were tested on three different tasks—one involving speed, another dexterity, and the third graphomotor skill. That excessive clumsiness is a feature in some children with reading disabilities has been observed by many teachers and has been confirmed by a number of researchers (110, 177).

TEST 6. *Pegboard Speed*

A two-sectioned pegboard was placed before the subjects, who were told to fill in, as quickly as possible, first the left and then the right side of the board.

TEST 7. *Tying a Knot*

The second test of fine motor skill required the children to tie a knot. This task was taken from the five-year level of the Stanford-Binet Intelligence Scale.

TEST 8. *Pencil Mastery*

The children's grasp and control of the pencil during graphomotor activities were observed. Teachers are familiar with the child who clutches the pencil in his fist, with the youngster who can barely hold the pencil, and with the one who presses so desperately hard that he tears the paper. Evalution of pencil control seemed of interest in terms of the relatively demanding graphomotor activities of first grade.

Laterality

TEST 9. *Hand Preference*

Consistency of hand preference during ball throwing, whittling, and pencil activities was noted. The test was designed to determine whether or not the child showed a clear-cut functional dominance of one hand over the other at kindergarten age.

Hand preference was the only aspect of lateralization explored, since, as has been demonstrated in Birch's and Belmont's (20) normative study, both eye and eye-hand consistency continue to be undetermined even at relatively high age levels.

That ambiguous lateralization, which is assumed to reflect poorly defined cerebral dominance (2, 254), is a concomitant of reading difficulties was postulated first by Orton (177). This hypothesis has, however, stimulated considerable controversy. Albert Harris (95) found insufficiently established hand preference in 40 per cent of the primary school children with reading difficulties (more than twice the proportion in an unselected group). However, recent researchers, such as Richard Coleman and Cynthia Deutsch (46) and Birch and Lillian Belmont (20), discovered no more ambilateral responses in older disabled readers than in their adequately performing peers.

Body Image

TEST 10. *Human-figure Drawing*

The children were asked to draw a picture of a boy or girl (depending on their sex). The drawings were evaluated solely according to cohesiveness and differentiation.

Bender (10) states that the body image is a Gestalt determined by laws of growth and development. That the maturational level of a child's human-figure drawing and his school achievement are significantly related has been demonstrated by a number of investigators (45, 207). Elizabeth Koppitz (143) found that a child's score on his human-figure drawing at the beginning of first grade was predictive of his reading level at the end of the year.[*]

[*] See Elizabeth Koppitz, *et al.*, "Prediction of First Grade School Achievement with the Bender Gestalt Test and Human Figure Drawings," *Journal of Clinical Psychology*, 15 (1959), 164–168.

Visual-perceptual Patterning

The two visual-perceptual performances investigated here were ability to discriminate figure from ground and visuomotor competence.

TEST 11. *Figure-ground Test*

A figure-ground test, adapted from Alfred Strauss and Laura Lehtinen (220), was administered.

That pulling out the "figure" from a strongly patterned ground is not an easy task is testified to by the fact that the well-known hidden figure puzzles present difficulties at young ages. Kindergarten children's visual-perceptual functioning is often fluid— nothing on the printed page stands out, and figure-ground difficulties have been observed to play a role in the reading disorders of elementary school children (59, 116, 208).

TEST 12. *Bender Visuo-Motor Gestalt Test*

Six of the nine designs were administered to all subjects. Criteria for evaluating the children's performance (evolved after discussion with Dr. Bender) included ability to respond to the essentials of the Gestalt and degree of differentiation (14).

Much time is spent in kindergarten helping children to recognize and to reproduce various forms and shapes. Such training serves to familiarize them with visuomotor experiences. The Bender Visuo-Motor Gestalt Test evaluates evolving competence in this area. Primitive and poorly integrated Bender Gestalten were found by Silver (207) and de Hirsch (109) to be characteristic of children with reading disabilities. That the Bender Visuo-Motor Gestalt Test predicts reading achievement as adequately as do reading readiness tests has been demonstrated by other studies (143, 215).

Auditory-perceptual Patterning

The fourteen tests administered in this area included five receptive-language and nine expressive-language dimensions. Receptive and expressive tests are listed separately only for purposes of presentation; it is recognized that the two language functions do in fact represent interrelated aspects of a multidimensional process (202).

Receptive-language Tests

TEST 13.   *Imitation of Tapped-out Patterns*

The children were required to imitate four increasingly complex tapped-out patterns.

Hardy (91) suggests that the ability to perceive, to process, and to reproduce sequences is a prerequisite for spoken and printed language. Some children experience difficulty even with nonverbal sequences. Ability to imitate tapped patterns, according to Stamback (219), increases with age; and Myklebust (168) maintains that this ability differentiates normal children from those with learning disorders.

TEST 14.   *Auditory Memory Span*

Repetition of two, three, and four nonsense syllables was required.

Virgil Anderson (3) observes that the ability to recall patterns of sounds and to organize them into language units matures slowly in a number of children. That the sequencing of auditory events plays a major part in oral-language functioning is well known; some children have a difficult time recalling nursery rhymes; they often fail to produce the correct number of syllables in spelling words. Some researchers comment on the relationship between auditory memory span and reading competence (192, 123).

TEST 15. *Auditory Discrimination*

Twenty alternate* word-pairs from Joseph Wepman's Auditory Discrimination Test (243) were presented, and the child was asked to judge whether they sounded the "same" or "different."

In this test the child has to perceive fine differences between sounds and to hold them in mind long enough to make comparisons between them. Appreciation of the meaning of words depends on such discrimination, which follows a maturational pattern (218, 244). In contrast to Margaret Byrne (33), who found few differences between good and poor readers on the Wepman Test, Deutsch (52) reported a significant association between auditory discrimination and reading.

TEST 16. *Word Recognition*

The children's performance on Lloyd Dunn's Peabody Picture Vocabulary Test (61) was used to judge comprehension of single nouns, verbs, and adverbs.

A child's mastery of printed words depends of necessity on his comprehension of these words when he hears them in conversation. In fact, Elmer Morgan (167), found a significant correlation between performance on a picture vocabulary test and reading achievement.

TEST 17. *Language Comprehension*

A simple story, appropriate for kindergarten age, was told to all subjects. Grasp of the gist of the story and comprehension of one spatial and two temporal concepts were evaluated. Insight into grammatical relationships and ability to process and retain

---

* The correlation coefficient between the split-half form and the entire test is .84, as reported by Wepman in a communication to the writers.

material heard are involved in this task. Both are of importance in reading, which requires the integration of content into an existing framework (187). A number of researchers (148, 165) found that comprehension tests administered at the beginning of first grade predicted reading success eight months later.

Expressive-language Tests

TEST 18. *Consonant Articulation*

Consonant articulation in spontaneous speech was measured by the Robert F. Hejna Developmental Articulation Test (102).

Articulatory competence depends on accurate perception and recall of word configurations, on adequate integration of fine-movement patterning of the speech mechanism, and on feedback. According to McCarthy (155) and Carroll (35), correct articulatory patterns are usually established by age six. Defective articulation may interfere with reading in several ways. A child who substitutes *th* for *s*, for instance, may confuse the words "sing" and "thing" when he meets them in print, and he may thus misinterpret the meaning of the sentence. Defective articulation, moreover, tends to interfere with the learning of phonics and has been reported to be a relatively frequent occurrence in children with reading difficulties (51, 239, 253).

TEST 19. *Articulatory Stability*

This competence was assessed by comparing the child's articulation on Hejna's test with his articulation during story telling.

There are children whose articulation of individual sounds is entirely acceptable, but whose speech disintegrates when they have to formulate complex ideas and the organizational load becomes too heavy.* In their clinical experience the authors have

---

* Frits Grewel (86) makes a distinction between defective articulation, on the one hand, and disturbance in the psycho-linguistic sphere, on the other. A child may, for instance, be able to produce a correct *f* or a *v*

found that children with disorganized and "cluttered" speech (4, 112, 241) almost invariably show spelling disabilities.

TEST 20. *Word Finding*

Naming the pictures from the Developmental Articulation Test was the basis for evaluating facility in evoking words.

A child's idiomatic speech may be adequate, but he may, nevertheless, be unable to evoke words in conversation or on presentation of pictures. Marked word-finding difficulties in poor readers have been reported by Muriel Langman (145) and others (122, 251).

TEST 21. *Story Organization*

The children were asked to tell *The Three Bears*, which is familiar to most and can be easily structured. Scoring was based on ability to get across the point of the story and to reproduce a number of relevant details.

In order for him to marshal events in a sequence, the child must have attained a fairly high level of inner language organization. Teachers know that some children are able to produce a vivid and logical account with a wealth of details, while others are either entirely unable to tell a story or tend to ramble on aimlessly. Weiner and Feldmann (240) found story telling to be predictive of end-of-first-grade reading performance.

TEST 22. *Number of Words*

The number of words used by the child during story telling was totaled.

McCarthy (154) believes that length of verbal responses is a relatively simple and objective measure of a child's level of spoken language.

---

in isolation, but he may fail to understand that the *f* is used in the singular form of "leaf," and that *v* is used for the plural. This type of error would indicate that he has not mastered the basic linguistic rules of his language.

Sentence Development

Maturity of children's sentence development was judged by analyzing taped recordings of each child's version of *The Three Bears*. McCarthy (154), Mildred Templin (227), and Sister Mary Shire (204) used as their basis for analysis children's spontaneous verbalizations during play, which may be more representative of a child's verbal output than the method used in the present study. Time limitations inherent in the administration of the long test battery, however, precluded the more spontaneous approach.

The number of utterances* obtained by using the story of *The Three Bears* ranged from 8 to 88, the mean being 28.87. This is comparable to the 25 utterances required by Ruth Strickland (221), but considerably below the minimum of 50 which, according to Frederick Darley and Kenneth Moll (49), constitutes a reliable index of a child's verbal development. In view of the fact that McCarthy (154) found the mean reliability coefficient between odd and even utterances (50 in all) to be .91, the writers felt justified in proceeding as described.

Level of sentence development, a facet of the child's language mastery, is related to a variety of factors: to environmental stimulation, as stressed by Deutsch (55); to the quality of the affect relationship between mother and child, as emphasized in the psychiatric literature (130); and to constitutional determinants, as discussed by Orton (175) and Langman (145). All of these seem to be valid and important. That maturational aspects are pertinent has been amply demonstrated by McCarthy (154), Shire (204), Templin (227), and Menyuk (164).

* Templin's (227) definition of "utterance" was used: "An utterance was considered completed if the child came to a complete stop, either letting the voice fall, giving interrogatory or exclamatory inflection, or indicating clearly that he did not intend to complete the sentence; if one single sentence was immediately followed by another with no pause for breath, or if the second statement was clearly subsidiary to the first."

Two facets of sentence development were measured. According to Shire (204), both differentiate between the best and the poorest readers.

TEST 23. *Sentence Elaboration*

The number of elaborated complex and compound sentences as defined by Templin (227) was the first measure of sentence development.

That some children use primitive sentence structures and others use complex ones is well known to kindergarten teachers. Strickland (221) found that the best readers used a significantly greater number of elaborated sentences than did the poorest readers.

TEST 24. *Number of Grammatical Errors*

For a second measure, two of Templin's (227) categories—incomplete sentences and grammatical errors—were combined.

At kindergarten age, children's mastery of the grammatical structure of the language varies strikingly. This variability is largely related to the way language is used in their homes. On the other hand, mastery of correct grammatical forms varies considerably within a given social milieu.

TEST 25. *Definitions*

The children were asked to define six words taken from the Stanford-Binet Intelligence Scale (Form L): "ball," "hat," "stove," (from year V) and "straw," "puddle," and "eyelash" (from year VI).

Piaget (186) questions the assumption that a child's ability to define words implies the beginning of conceptualization. He feels, rather, that it reflects the level of the child's linguistic maturity. Artley (5) states that ". . . any limitation in word meaning . . . would have a bearing on reading ability."

TEST 26. *Categories*

The children were requested to produce generic names for three clusters of words.

The child's ability to determine whether a number of objects belong together in terms of the features they have in common reflects the beginning of generalization.

Reading Readiness Tests

It was recognized that training at home and at school heavily influences performance on reading readiness tests. However, most kindergarten teachers realize that some children are better able to respond to such training than are others.

TEST 27. *Letter Copying*

Copying letters requires a modicum of perceptual organization and eye-hand coordination. Young children copy letters much in the way they draw a picture. However, copying letters is a more demanding task than drawing, since the child has to focus attention on the direction, form, and size of abstract shapes.

TEST 28. *Name Writing*

The children were told to write their first names. Name writing is a relatively highly integrated performance compared to letter copying. Not only does the child lack a model when he writes his name, but he has to acquire a feeling for the orientation of the configuration of the whole name.

TEST 29. *Letter Naming*

Six letters of the alphabet were exposed and the children were asked to name them.

It has been shown that ability to name letters at the beginning of first grade is highly predictive of reading achievement at the end of the year (62, 166, 206).

TEST 30.   *The Horst Test*

This test forms one part of the first version of a larger reading readiness test, constructed by Horst.* Goins (82) found that matching sequences of objects and shapes is positively related to subsequent reading achievement. However, because, according to Harris, only the ability to match letters is important for reading (96), only that part of the Horst Test was used here which requires the child to match two- and three-letter sequences. (See Appendix II.)

Matching of letter sequences is a difficult task at kindergarten age, not only because of the abstract nature of the stimuli, but also because it requires the holding in mind of two- and three-letter sequences.

TESTS 31 *and* 32.   *Gates Matching and Rhyming Subtests*

Abbreviated versions of the Gates Matching and Rhyming subtests were administered.

TESTS 33, 34, *and* 35.   *Word Recognition (I and II) and Reproduction of Words Previously Taught (Jansky)*

At the beginning of the session, the child was shown how to read two words, "boy" and "train," and was told to copy them from a model. At the end of the two-hour session, the child was required: To select, from a pack of cards presented successively, the words "boy" and "train"; to identify the same words when

---

* This test, constructed by Dr. Maria Horst and used for research purposes in Holland (87) and France (212), is in the process of being re-edited and changed and is being considered for use, in its new version, by the New York City Public Schools. (Horst, Maria. "Het Onderzoek van de Leesrijpheid bij Zesjarige Kinderen," *Nederlands Tijdschrift voor de Psychologie,* 13 (1958), 229–258.)

they were exposed with eight others on the table; and to write from memory as much of the two words as he was able to recall.

Sylvia Gavel (77) and Alice Nicholson (171) found that recognition of words taught, as measured at the beginning of first grade, is predictive of reading competence at the end of the school year.

Style

It has long been recognized that a child's style of attacking a task is an important factor in his scholastic achievement. An attempt was therefore made to evaluate two categories impressionistically—ego strength and work attitude. These categories were included because it was assumed that a child with considerable ego strength and a positive attitude toward work would be better able to compensate for perceptuomotor deficits than one whose approach to work was lacking in vigor.

TEST 36.   *Ego Strength*

A clinical evaluation of ego strength was attempted. The concept of ego strength was mentioned by Ives Hendrick (103) in 1934: It is described by him as ". . . a certain capacity for fighting difficulties . . . grit." The child with adequate ego strength would be ". . . in full possession of his organismic energies. . . ." (248). Sibylle Escalona and Grace Heider (64) found that assessment of available energy enhanced the reliability of prediction.

TEST 37.   *Work Attitude*

The extent to which the child was able to invest energy in a goal-directed way was assessed. Work attitude was described as "good" only if the child used his energy in the service of the task.

Profile

Immediately after concluding the kindergarten test series the writers wrote a short profile of each child, in which they summarized their impressions of his over-all functioning, as well as of his specific weakness and strength. These profiles supplemented the statistical data with pertinent clinical observations, and were added to after each contact with the child.

TESTS ADMINISTERED AT END OF GRADE I

At the end of the first grade, all children were tested in writing [Frank Freeman's Zaner-Bloser Test (69)] and reading (the Gates Sentence and Paragraph and the Gray Oral Reading tests).*

TESTS ADMINISTERED AT END OF GRADE II

Writing Test

A series of four sentences was dictated. The subjects were free to choose between printing and cursive writing.

Writing to dictation presupposes grasp of meaning. By the time a child reaches the end of his second year in school, he should be able to some extent to withdraw attention from the writing act; the visual and auditory image should fuse with the movement Gestalt of the word. Children may fail in writing for different reasons: They may be unable to recall letter shapes (ideational agraphia), or they may have difficulty with the execution of movements (motor dysgraphia). Severe disorders of writing have been extensively treated by Hermann and H. Voldby (107).

Reading Tests

The Gates Advanced Primary and the Gray Oral Reading tests were administered.

* Findings related to Grade I tests are occasionally referred to in Chapters 5, 6, and 8.

Spelling Test

The children were given the spelling subtest of the Metropolitan Achievement Test, Primary II Battery. In spelling, the child must recall not only the visual configuration of the whole word, but also its internal design. Beyond visual recall, spelling requires ability to appreciate the auditory features of the word. The youngster who perceives the word "interesting" as "inersting," for example, will misspell the word.

Kindergarten Tests Readministered

At the end of second grade, four items from the kindergarten test battery were readministered, so as to gain an impression of the ongoing changes in the children's performance and behavior. Test items repeated were: Behavioral Patterning, Hand Preference, Bender Visuo-Motor Gestalt Test, and Auditory Discrimination Test.

Profile

Finally, the child's style of approach was reassessed at this level. His specific approach to reading was noted. These observations served as a basis for comparison with the profiles formulated at kindergarten age.

3

Procedures, Findings, and Discussion

•

PROCEDURES

In order to identify those kindergarten tests that might serve as potential predictors of end-of-second-grade performance, coefficients were computed measuring the correlation between each kindergarten test and a summary measure of silent and oral end-of-second-grade reading achievement. Analogous coefficients were computed for spelling and writing scores. Those kindergarten tests that yielded significant correlation coefficients were retained as potential predictors. All others were dropped from further consideration. The same procedure was followed for selected background variables.

Multiple regression and correlation, the best methods available for the construction of predictive instruments, could not be used in this study because the data did not meet the assumption that the scores on each test be normally distributed. On about half of the kindergarten tests, the distribution of scores was markedly skewed. For the same reason, the Pearsonian product moment coefficient of correlation was not appropriate.

The coefficients of correlation selected were Kendall's tau-beta (134) coefficient and the d_{yx} (217) coefficient. These are coefficients of rank-order correlation which are independent of a normal distribution and related assumptions. Although not as powerful as multiple regression, and not suited to show the relative contributions of individual items, these coefficients satisfactorily identify the best predictive tests. As in the case of parametric correlation coefficients, a value of .00 indicates no relationship at all between the variables compared, while a value of 1.00 indicates a perfect correlation.

OVER-ALL READING PERFORMANCE INDEX (ORP INDEX)

To compute the correlations between the kindergarten tests and end-of-second-grade performance, a single measure of reading competence was developed, combining the Gates Advanced Primary and the Gray Oral Reading tests (see Appendix Table I-1). Although these two instruments are not of equal difficulty, the differences between scores were not pronounced, and combining them seemed justifiable because of the highly significant correlation (tau-beta = .60) between the Gates and the Gray measures. Because the present investigation was concerned with reading competence in general, rather than with the separate skills of silent and oral reading, a single index seemed preferable.

It should be understood, however, that any statement made in these pages concerning the ORP Index is applicable, without substantial modification, to the Gray and Gates tests separately as well.

FINDINGS

Correlation of the Thirty-seven Kindergarten Tests with End-of-Second-Grade Scores

Among the thirty-seven kindergarten tests, nineteen were significantly related to the ORP Index, twenty to spelling, and sixteen to writing performance (see Appendix Table I-2).

Kindergarten tests significantly related to end-of-second-grade reading achievement were Behavioral Control, Pencil Use, Human-figure Drawing, Bender Visuo-Motor Gestalt Test, Tapped-out Patterns, Wepman Auditory Discrimination Test, Story Organization, Number of Words Used, Categories, Name Writing, Letter Naming, Horst Reversals Test, Word Matching, Word Rhyming, Word Recognition I and II, Word Reproduction, Ego Strength, and Work Attitude.

Kindergarten tests significantly related to end-of-second-grade spelling performance were Behavioral Control, Pegboard Speed, Human-figure drawing, Bender Visuo-Motor Gestalt Test, Tapped-out Patterns, Wepman Auditory Discrimination Test, Peabody Picture Vocabulary Test, Story Organization, Number of Words Used, Categories, Name Writing, Letter Copying, Letter Naming, Horst Reversals Test, Word Matching, Word Recognition I and II, Word Reproduction, Ego Strength, and Work Attitude.

Kindergarten tests significantly related to end-of-second-grade writing were Behavioral Control, Pegboard Speed, Pencil Use, Bender Visuo-Motor Gestalt Test, Number of Words Used, Categories, Name Writing, Copying of Letters, Letter Naming, Horst Reversals Test, Word Matching, Word Recognition I and II, Word Reproduction, Ego Strength, and Work Attitude.

The d_{yx} coefficients for these correlations appear lower than the correlations between predictive variables and reading performance reported in other studies. Among the coefficients reported which differed significantly from zero, values ranged from .23 to .56. These relatively low coefficients are in all probability due to a statistical artifact: The d_{yx} coefficient is characteristically lower numerically than the corresponding Pearsonian coefficient for the same set of data.* In other words, had the present data

---

* For purposes of comparison, Pearsonian coefficients corresponding to the d_{yx} coefficients were computed between three of the kindergarten tests

warranted use of the Pearsonian coefficient, levels of correlation would probably have been of the same order numerically as those reported in other predictive studies.

Correlation of Background Variables with End-of-Second-Grade Performance

None of the ten background variables pertaining to *family history and verbal stimulation* was significantly correlated with the ORP Index, with spelling, or with writing (see Appendix Table I-3).

When *IQ* was treated in the same way as the thirty-seven kindergarten tests, as a potential predictor, the relationship with end-of-second-grade reading achievement was significant at the 5 per cent level of confidence ($d_{yx} = .31$). The correlation between IQ and spelling was not significant ($d_{yx} = .19$); that between IQ and writing was negligible ($d_{yx} = .05$).

As a next step the possible contribution of intelligence to the correlations that had been found to be statistically significant was assessed (see Appendix Table I-4). On only one of the nineteen tests (Letter Naming) did IQ appear to "account for" the significant association with reading competence two and a half years later.[*]

Since differences between *boys and girls* in rate of maturation may have affected prediction, separate coefficients of correlation were computed for boys and girls, for those nineteen tests that were potential predictors. The findings (see Appendix Table I-5)

---

on which the distribution of scores was not overly skewed and the Over-all Reading Performance Index. The results were as follows:

Correlation Between ORP and:	d_{yx}	Pearsonian
Letter naming	.54	.65
Bender Visuo-Motor Gestalt Test	.44	.56
Human-figure drawing	.23	.29

[*] Our reservations as to the appropriateness of "accounting" for IQ are discussed in Chapter 6.

indicate that while three tests predicted about equally well for both, and two predicted better for boys, the overwhelming majority of tests were much better predictors for girls.

Girls' and boys' performance at the end of second grade was compared next (see Appendix Table I-6).* Although girls' achievement was superior to that of boys at this level, the differences were not statistically significant.

When *chronological* age at first-grade entrance was treated in the same way as the thirty-seven kindergarten tests, the correlation with end-of-second-grade ORP Index was significant at the 5 per cent level of confidence ($d_{yx} = .23$).

A comparison of the end-of-second-grade performance of *Negro and Caucasian* children showed that the Caucasian children achieved higher scores on reading, spelling, and writing tests; however, only in the case of spelling did the difference between groups reach statistical significance (see Appendix I, Table I-7).

DISCUSSION OF FINDINGS

The fact that intelligence did not basically account for the correlations between single perceptuomotor and oral-language tests and second-grade achievement, was one of the most interesting findings.

It is true that IQ, when treated as a single predictor, was significantly related to achievement two and a half years later; however, IQ ranked only twelfth among predictive measures; eleven other kindergarten tests were better predictors of subsequent reading. Furthermore, the correlation between IQ and spelling was very low, which supports our clinical experience that severe spelling disabilities are highly specific and cannot easily be compensated for by intelligence.

That most tests predicted better for *girls* than for *boys* may

* Details about "critical scores" for all comparisons: sex, age, race, prematurely versus maturely born subjects, are available.

have been due in part to the fact that, as a group, the girls were somewhat older. Even when age was taken into account, however, the predictions remained higher for girls—perhaps, and this is clearly speculative, because the developmental course of girls is more consistent.

The significantly poorer spelling of the *Negro* as compared to the *Caucasian* children may possibly be related to the inferior auditory discrimination of the Negro youngsters. An inspection of the data did show lower auditory discrimination in this group. Whether poor auditory discrimination among Negro children is related to differences in dialect, to social class, or to both, are questions which cannot be answered on the basis of the data.

The virtual absence of associations between second-grade achievement and *family history of language and handedness* might be attributable to lack of accurate information. Charles Wenar (242) refers to the unreliability of parental reports. Orton (175) and his pupils, who were strongly impressed with positive family histories in cases of reading failure, dealt with middle and upper middle class parents, who were presumably more interested in and better informed about academic achievement and handedness in their background than were parents in the group studied here, who belonged to a lower socio-economic stratum. Furthermore, most previous investigations, unlike the present one, drew on populations of disabled readers, not on unselected groups of children—which may explain the discrepancy in the findings.

Contrary to expectations, no significant correlations were found between end-of-second-grade achievement and various measures of *environmental* stimulation. The only correlation that approached significance was the children's response to television. Since television presumably plays a major role in the parents' own lives, their observations in this area may have been more accurate and complete than were those that dealt with storytelling and the children's response to it. The relative homogeneity of the children's background may also have reduced the probability of significant correlations.

Our expectations that certain *kindergarten tests* would be predictive of performance two and a half years later were based primarily on clinical experience and on reports by other researchers. In the following pages the findings are examined in the light of these expectations.

It may be of interest to discuss first those tests that *failed* to be predictive:

By the time our children had reached kindergarten age, gross motor skills, such as hopping, throwing, and balancing were probably too well established in the group as a whole to serve as a basis for differentiation. It is quite likely that a year or two earlier, the same tests would have differentiated between subjects. To some extent, this may have been true also for the figure-ground discrimination test, which was probably too easy for the kindergarten children. A more demanding task of the same type might have differentiated better at the kindergarten level.

The data demonstrated that ill-defined lateralization at kindergarten age did not preclude adequate or better reading competence at the end of second grade. We believe that differentiation between hands is related to maturation. [Antonio Subirana's findings (222) of more mature electroencephalograms in strongly right-handed as against ambidextrous and left-handed children would support this hypothesis.] However, those two-thirds of our subjects who had settled early on a preferred hand did not read better than those who had not.

Next to be examined will be those tests that were *positively* associated with later performance:

It was not surprising to find that *hyperactive, distractible,* and *disinhibited* behavior was positively associated with subsequent scores. It is true that the eleven children who, at kindergarten age, had been at the mercy of a multitude of environmental stimuli had acquired better controls by the end of the second grade. Nevertheless, a degree of restlessness and a low frustration threshold continued to interfere with performance.

The fact that Pegboard Speed, a relatively sensitive test of *fine motor control*, was significantly related to writing had been expected; it was remarkable, on the other hand, that Pegboard Speed was associated with spelling. This lends support to early statements by Orton (177), who drew attention to psychomotor lags in children with reading and spelling disorders.

Graphomotor ability showed a fairly high correlation with reading and writing two and one-half years later. Difficulties with pencil management are occasionally found in children who are skillful in manipulating objects like puzzles or models. The fact that an activity like name writing was associated with reading competence seems to show that in name writing verbal symbolic factors, in addition to motoric ones, are involved.

That the ability of a young child to project the image of his own body onto paper enters to some extent into his later reading and spelling achievement is testified to by the weak but statistically significant correlation between early *human-figure drawings* and the ORP Index. That the ability to draw a human figure is not primarily a motor task is suggested by the fact that this performance was not significantly associated with writing. A child's body image results from integration of his proprioceptive, sensorimotor, emotional, and social experiences. It does not actually represent a figure seen, but reflects rather the child's awareness of his own body, its parts, and their relationship to each other. Birch and Belmont (20) think it possible that defects in body schema and praxis enter into reading failure. Such defects may be reflected in the human-figure drawings of preschool children.

The *Bender Visuo-Motor Gestalt Test* ranked near the top among tests that correlated significantly with end-of-second-grade achievement. Silver (207) stresses the importance of the integrative functions in this task—visual stimuli are sifted through the experience and organic matrix of the individual and are thus integrated. Children's copies of the Bender Gestalten vary at different maturational and growth levels; ability to cross wavy lines and to cope with diagonals and corners, for instance, matures at six to eight years, around the time the child enters first grade. The findings in this study justify the use of the shortened version of this test for predictive purposes at kindergarten age.

Five *oral language* tests—two in the receptive and three in the expressive area—predicted subsequent achievement. Oral and printed forms of language extend along a time-space continuum. In reading, space is used to indicate time; the printed word is a time chart of sounds (56). The literature, beginning with Orton (177), is filled with statements that refer to the close interrelationship between auditory-perceptual and oral-language deficits, on the one hand, and reading difficulties, on the other (25, 108). There is, however, according to McCarthy (155), little agreement as to the extent and nature of this relationship. It was of interest that one nonverbal test that involved temporal organization— Imitation of Tapped-out Patterns—showed a fairly high predictive potential. That two other tests in the *receptive-language* area— Auditory Discrimination and the Peabody Picture Vocabulary Test—were significantly associated with end-of-second-grade scores was less noteworthy, since both are verbal measures.

Among the *expressive-language* tests administered at the kindergarten level, Number of Words Used in a Story proved to be by far the best predictor. Performance on this task varied to an extraordinary degree—the number of words used ranged from 54 to 594. Richness of verbal output, whether related to environmental stimulation or to inherent linguistic endowment or to both, is apparently an excellent prognostic sign. Organization of a Story, which requires ability to integrate details into a mean-ingful whole, was another test that showed a statistically signi-ficant association with end-of-second-grade achievement.

All *reading readiness* tests except one (Letter Copying) were predictive of later performance. These tests primarily involve visual perception. According to Gibson (81), visual perception starts as a crudely differentiated and grossly selective process. The child learns only slowly to identify critical features in a given configuration. Most reading readiness tests, since they require the child to respond to abstract forms, that is to say, to letters and words, demand a high level of visual-perceptual maturity.[*] It is not surprising, therefore, that nearly all reading readiness tasks showed significant correlations with later achievement meas-ures.

It will be seen that tests that were found to be predictive were not confined to one specific area of kindergarten functioning. Reading readiness tests such as Word Matching and Name Writ-ing measure, of course, performances that are similar to those involved in the reading and writing process itself. However, the Human-figure drawing and the Bender Gestalt tests were also predictive, although they assess skills that have no apparent or direct relation to reading. Both these tests, like reading, writing, and spelling, require the ability to organize parts of a Gestalt into a meaningful whole; in other words, they call for a relatively high degree of integrative competence. Alan Ross (196) defines integration as that function of the organism which combines and relates discrete cues and makes a unified response possible. In our opinion the predictive efficacy of the tests depended not on the specific skills involved, but on the degree to which they meas-ured integrative ability. If this ability is weak at kindergarten age, it augurs poorly for reading and spelling at the end of

[*] Tests like Marianne Frostig's (73) are designed to quantify visual-perceptual competence and maturation.

second grade, since at that stage a relatively high level of integration is required. By the time a child has reached the eighth year of life, he must, according to Birch and Belmont (21), be able to use information gained from both auditory and visual clues— in other words, he must be able to integrate intersensory information, a very demanding task.

It is noteworthy that in this study positive correlations were found between *ego strength* and *work attitude,* on the one hand, and all achievement measures, on the other. Difficulties with integration are assumed to account for defects in ego strength. It is regrettable that our investigation could not explore the fascinating interrelationships between integrative lags on the physiological level and those found on the level of ego organization.

4
The Predictive Index

◆

The construction of a predictive index for the use of schools was a major goal of our study. This index was to consist of those tests which, in combination, would most effectively identify high-risk children. (That the index would also serve to single out average or high achievers was considered to be of secondary importance.)

The Predictive Index discussed in the following pages was constructed to forecast reading and spelling but not writing achievement. The correlation between writing and reading, although significant, was low (tau-beta=.38), while that between spelling and reading at the end of the second grade was very high (tau-beta=.74). Many kindergarten tests showed significant correlations with *both* reading and spelling performance two and a half years later. Since it thus seems that the abilities underlying reading and spelling are closely related, the construction of an index useful for predicting both achievements appeared to be justified. (We believe that the correlations between reading and spelling would be lower in the higher grades; many older children seen in clinical practice "catch on" to reading, yet continue to fail in spelling.)

In deciding which of the kindergarten tests were most suitable for inclusion in a predictive index, the following three criteria were used:

1. Each test should exhibit relatively high and statistically significant levels of correlation with the ORP Index and the Metropolitan Spelling Test scores at the end of the second grade.

2. Each test should show a score distribution free of characteristics such as excessive skewness that might render its association with end-of-second-grade reading and spelling suspect.

3. Each test should differentiate clearly between average or better readers and spellers and below-average or poor readers and spellers.

Thirteen kindergarten tests satisfied all of these criteria. They were: Pencil Use, Bender Visuo-Motor Gestalt, Wepman Auditory Discrimination Test, Number of Words, Categories, Horst Reversals, Gates Word Matching, Word Recognition I and II, Word Reproduction, Imitation of Tapped-out Patterns, Name Writing, and Letter Naming. On the basis of an analysis of correlations among these thirteen predictors, varying combinations of from three to ten tests each—over one hundred such combinations in all—were tried experimentally. Indexes were compared to determine which combination would best identify those children who subsequently failed.

A number of trial indexes seemed promising. The index chosen consisted of ten tests, listed below, each of which contributed to the effectiveness of the instrument as a whole (see Appendix II for instructions and scoring).

> Pencil Use
> Bender Visuo-Motor Gestalt Test
> Wepman Auditory Discrimination Test
> Number of Words Used in a Story
> Categories
> Horst Reversals Test
> Gates Word Matching Test

Word Recognition I
Word Recognition II
Word Reproduction

It is, of course, possible that after validation procedures have been completed, the Predictive Index may be modified in some respects. Letter Naming, for instance, might be added because it is a promising test. It should be recognized that performance in this area is partly dependent on prior training. This test was not used for the Predictive Index here because it had been administered to only half the sample.

A given child's Predictive Index score was determined by the following procedure: The score level that best discriminated between the failing readers and the rest of the children was computed for each test; the child's Predictive Index score was simply the number of tests on which he scored at or above the critical score level. (The critical score levels for each of the ten tests are listed in Appendix III and Table III-1.)

The effectiveness of the Predictive Index in identifying failing readers or spellers among the children studied here is shown in Appendix Table I-8. Index scores from zero to 3 correctly identified ten of the eleven children (91 per cent) who failed reading or spelling tests at the end of second grade. However, the Index also picked up four "false positives"—children who scored 3 or lower on the index, but who nevertheless passed end-of-second-grade tests. It seems that in order to increase the chances of identifying virtually all failing children, it is necessary to throw out a large net, as it were, one which will inevitably pick up some adequate readers. Such an approach is, of course, consistent with public health practices which provide preventive measures for large populations in order to eliminate the possibility of overlooking potential risks.

A careful consideration of the individual children for whom the index predicted incorrectly is in order—not to "explain away" inaccurate forecasts but to portray the kind of children for whom predictions are likely to go awry.

There was, first, the single failing reader missed by the Predictive Index. This boy's performance at kindergarten age, while not outstanding, was at any rate acceptable. He was a little doubt-ridden and quite critical of himself, but so were many other subjects. He was young on entering first grade (5 years, 11 months), but so were other children who did not fail. He changed teachers during the first grade, and some of his classmates in his school in Harlem were reported by the teacher to be disturbed; however, he was not the only chronologically young subject in this study who entered a none-too-well-organized class. It is of course possible that it was the accumulation of adverse factors, each inconclusive in itself, that resulted in failure. In any case, we have no really compelling explanation for the fact that this boy, against expectations, failed second-grade tests.

Of the four children whom the index placed in the "failing" category but who nevertheless passed achievement tests at the end of second grade, one, a girl with poor eyesight, had been fitted for glasses only a day or two before her kindergarten interview. The examiner's comment in the chart reads: "Her poor visuomotor performance may be a residual from the time when her vision was defective." This girl, as well as one other child, a boy, had, in fact, failed all reading tests at the end of *first* grade; both, for different reasons, had been slow starters. We believe that the girl will do well at school in the long run, while the boy, who barely passed at the end of his second grade, may very well have difficulties later on.

Of the remaining two children in the "false positive" category, one was just six years old when he entered first grade; at kindergarten age, his auditory-perceptual and oral-language tools had been very poor. Dramatic developmental spurts in the interval between kindergarten and the end of second grade may well have accounted for the inaccurate forecast. Such sudden spurts in maturation probably constitute the real pitfalls in predictions of this kind. The fourth child in the same category was quite a disturbed youngster. He vomited each morning before going to school, and for this reason was kept home for long periods of time. He did poorly on the initial tests, and we do not know why, in spite of his continuing disturbance, he performed so much better later on.

Unfortunately, limitations in time and funds did not permit the collection of many pertinent data, such as significant events in the child's life between kindergarten and the end of second grade. The quality of teaching in the first two grades, frequent changes in school placement, major upheavals in the home—all enter into academic achievement and thus are bound to influence the accuracy of prediction. In spite of these limitations, the Predictive Index effectively identified at kindergarten age the overwhelming majority of children who failed at the end of their second year at school.

5

The Failing Readers

◆

Our primary goal was the early identification of academic high-risk children. So as to help the teachers in the early recognition of such youngsters, we examined the kindergarten protocols of those children who showed massive reading and spelling difficulties at the end of the second grade.

A review of their performance and behavior at kindergarten age revealed a characteristic flavor not conveyed by the test scores. In the following chapter we attempt to describe these children clinically. Furthermore, in order to highlight their particular pattern of dysfunctions, we will compare the group of failing children with two other groups—the "Slow Starters," who had trouble with reading in the beginning but later overcame their initial lags, and the "Superior Achievers," who excelled from the start.

The Failing Reader group consisted of eight subjects whose achievement at the end of the second grade made up the lowest 15 per cent among the children tested. All of these failing children had scored zero on the Gray Oral Reading Test* at the end of the first grade. Five of them again received a score of zero

* The Gray Oral Reading Test was chosen because it is more stringent than the Gates in that it does not allow the child to guess from pictorial clues.

a year later; the highest rating among the remaining three children was nine months below the norm. It is evident, therefore, that these subjects had in no way caught up by the end of their second year in the elementary grades.

The group consisted of three Negro and five Caucasian children. In all but one case, one or both parents had attended high school. Seven of the eight children had been enrolled in kindergarten; at the end of the second grade, the eight failing subjects were attending eight different schools—three parochial and five public. IQs in the group ranged from 94 to 116.

Six of the eight failing children were boys. The preponderance of boys among children with difficulties in reading and related language skills has been discussed by many researchers and has been interpreted in the light of the particular theoretical position of each. For example, Jerome Kagan (125) believes that boys do not find activities in the primary grades to be congruent with their masculine role. On the other hand, J. M. Tanner's (224) observation that, around the age of six, males lag twelve months behind girls in skeletal age points to important physiological reasons for the inferior academic performance of boys. Bentzen (18) believes that learning problems in boys may be the response of the immature organism to the demands of a society which fails to make appropriate provision for the biological age differential between girls and boys. Emmett Betts (19) and Bryant (28) all speak of boys' lesser capacity to mature smoothly.

Five of the Failing Readers were unusually small. In the absence of information as to parental stature, it would be hazardous to generalize from this observation. Olson (173) concludes, on the basis of his investigations, that biophysical and educational age are related and that reading is ". . . in obscure ways tied to the entire developmental process." Maria Simon (213) reports that her failing subjects tended to show up as "immature" on a battery of anthropomorphic indexes. Robert Karlin (128) found a small but statistically significant relation between carpal development and reading ability in first grade. Skeletal age was retarded in sixteen poor readers in Ralph House's (117) sample of fifty-three first graders. Ilg and Ames, (118) who emphasize the importance of developmental age in the assessment of first-grade readiness, draw attention to the relationship between teething schedule and school achievement.

Clinically, it was clear from the start that the Failing Readers were unable to respond to the testing in a purposeful and organized way, in spite of the fact that each was examined individually, a procedure that usually makes it easier for the subject to attend to the task at hand. Five of the Failing Readers were markedly hyperactive, distractible, impulsive, and disinhibited; they needed many opportunities to move around the room, and became resentful when they were required to sit still. One boy, for instance, asked repeatedly to be allowed to "dance," by which he meant to jump up and down. Three of the children presented the opposite picture in terms of activity level: They were hypoactive, had difficulty maintaining a sitting posture, and tended to slump. Their throwing was hypotonic; some of them could hardly hold a pencil. Both hyper- and hypoactive youngsters showed a considerable tendency to fatigue. Toward the end of the testing session, they were altogether unable to function.

"Infantile" was the term used in the profiles for five of the Failing Readers. Whining, crying, and an excessive need for candy were among the behaviors subsumed under this term. Two of the children were able to complete the testing only after they had been taken on the examiner's lap.

The Failing Readers did not show more concomitant movements than did the children in the other two groups, nor was their gross motor performance particularly deviant. On the other hand, their fine manual control was poor: they were slow at inserting pegs into a board; the large majority, moreover, had severe difficulties with graphomotor tasks.

Contrary to expectations, ambilateral responses were no more frequent among the Failing Readers than among the Slow Starters and the Superior Achievers. Differences were found, however, in body-image concept. While the Failing Readers' figure drawings were not bizarre, they were strikingly crude and undifferentiated.

The auditory-perceptual and oral-language tools of the Failing Readers, furthermore, were decidedly inferior to those of the remaining subjects. The Failing Readers' auditory discrimination, for instance, seemed to be extraordinarily diffuse; in fact, several of the children insisted that most of the word-pairs presented in the discrimination test sounded exactly alike. Their recognition vocabulary was limited; they showed subtle gaps in language comprehension, as evidenced by their inability to grasp the essential parts of a story and to place them in proper relation to the whole. They had equally striking difficulties with the expressive aspects of language. While only two subjects presented severe articulatory defects or disturbances in the rhythmic flow of speech, the stories of five others were relatively primitive, lacking in cohesiveness, and poorly integrated. Severe word-finding difficulties were characteristic for these children; shown a picture of a stove and asked to name it, they would produce the word "kitchen-thing." Several children were unable to provide generic terms for groups of words. In short, the Failing Readers showed not only more numerous but also more severe deficits in both the receptive and the expressive aspects of language than did the Slow Starters and the Superior Achievers.

On visual-perceptual tasks, the Failing Readers did poorly. They had trouble "pulling out" the figure from a strongly structured ground on the test specifically constructed for this purpose, and they frequently failed to respond to the "critical" configurations in some of the reading readiness tests. They had marked difficulties, moreover, in copying the Bender Visuo-Motor Gestalten. In many cases their designs flowed into each other, testifying to the plastic and fluid character of their perceptuomotor experiences. Most of their copies, furthermore, were strikingly crude and undifferentiated; and some showed evidence of perceptual fragmentation.

Of all the kindergarten tests administered, reading readiness tests were the most difficult, perhaps because of the relatively abstract nature of the tasks. The Failing Readers showed very inferior performance in all of these activities. For instance, when asked to select from among a number of words one that had been exposed earlier, the children responded as if the printed configurations were simply a jumble of meaningless designs, all looking more or less alike and lacking in distinct physiognomic features. It is true that success or failure on certain reading readiness tests, such as Name Writing, Letter Identification, and Letter Copying, depends largely on previous exposure and experience. The same cannot be said, however, for the Reversal, the Matching, and the Word Reproduction tests, which do not seem to be *directly* influenced by training. It thus appears that the Failing Readers' poor showing on these tests was related to some inherent characteristics in the children themselves.

One can do little more than speculate as to the nature of this characteristic. That important differences existed between the Failing Readers and the other children, and that, as a result, the Failing Readers were identifiable at an early age, is borne out by the fact that we were able to predict academic failure in seven of the eight children under discussion.*

THE SLOW STARTERS

The group of Slow Starters consisted of four boys and four

---

* We refer here to our *clinical* predictions, as opposed to the correlations between kindergarten tests and end-of-second-grade performance scores. These particular predictions were formulated immediately after the administration of the kindergarten tests, on the basis of a combination of clinical impressions and test performance.

girls. Like the Failing Readers, they had scored zero on the Gray
Oral Reading Tests at the end of the first grade. Unlike the Failing Readers, however, the Slow Starters achieved at the expected
level at the end of the second grade. It is evident, therefore, that
at least in reading, their difficulties were transient and that, with
continued growth and instruction, they had learned to cope.

The Slow Starters' kindergarten protocols did not report hyperactivity, disinhibition, or distractibility. By kindergarten age these
children had apparently achieved a measure of behavioral control.
Compared with the human-figure drawings of the Failing Readers,
those of the Slow Starters were less primitive; their auditory
perception was less diffuse, and their stories less impoverished
and fragmentary. They had no trouble with figure-ground discrimination and the organization of the visual field. The Slow
Starters, in short, did fairly well on less complex tasks, and began
to fail only when they moved on to activities that called for more
highly integrated performances, such as the Bender Gestalt, Story
Organization, and most reading readiness tests. One might say,
therefore, that at the kindergarten level, the Slow Starters' perceptuomotor experiences were better organized and their central
nervous system (CNS) patterning less primitive than that of the
Failing Readers, but that in tests that required more differentiated
and more highly integrated responses, their real difficulties became
apparent.

Up to a point these difficulties persisted. While all eight Slow
Starters managed to pass reading tests at the end of the second
grade, the spelling achievement of half the group remained inferior.

The uneven maturation pattern of the Slow Starters made clinical predictions for these children far more hazardous than for the
subjects in the other groups. In fact, our predictions for the Slow
Starters (as opposed to the predictive index scores) were not
much better than might have been expected had they been made
by chance.

THE SUPERIOR ACHIEVERS

The Superior Achievers' performance constituted the highest 15 per cent in the general sample, both in reading and in spelling. At the end of the second grade, their reading ranged from one to two years above the norm. The group consisted of two boys and six girls. When they entered first grade, all the Superior Achievers were older—6 years, 5 months or above—than were the Failing Readers and the Slow Starters, thus apparently confirming Hall's (89) and Ilg and Ames' (118) findings of generally better achievement among overage pupils than among underage ones.* The Superior Achievers were specifically described in the protocols as "mature" or "physically well developed."

This group's kindergarten functioning was uniformly excellent. It is true that the children showed isolated drops in performance, but these occasional lapses were offset by top scores in all other areas. The Superior Achievers displayed advanced linguistic ability: The most complex sentence structures were found in the stories of the children in this group. Most impressive was the Superior Achievers' high-order performance on reading readiness tests. Viewed as a whole, the Superior Achievers' preschool functioning was so much better than that of the other children that success at the end of the second grade could be predicted clinically, without any reservation whatsoever.

GROUP COMPARISONS

The following chart shows the number of children in each of the three groups—Failing Readers, Slow Starters, and Superior Achievers—who failed representative kindergarten tests. It is clear from this chart that the Failing Readers' kindergarten functioning was inferior to that of the children in the other two groups.

* For the exception, see the children discussed in Chapter 9.

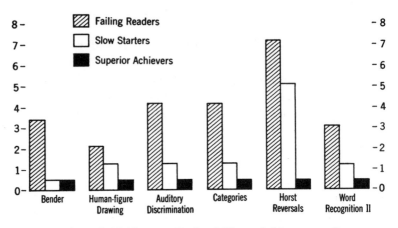

Number of Children in Each of Three Achievement Groups
Who Failed on Representative Kindergarten Tests

The kindergarten protocols of the three reading groups as they
ranged from failing to passing to superior show a progression
from diffuse and primitive responses among the Failing Readers
to differentiated and sharply defined ones among the Superior
Achievers. Edward French (70) states that there are children
who have trouble stabilizing at high levels of perceptual organization. The Failing Readers' perceptuomotor and linguistic responses were strikingly unstable. As do chronologically younger
children, they functioned at a primitive and undifferentiated level.
Their fragmented human-figure drawings, their poorly synthesized
Bender designs, their inability to organize parts of a story into a
meaningful whole, suggested a relatively low level of integrative
competence. (See illustrations on pages 53 and 54.)

It was not, however, failure on any *single* task that distinguished
the Failing Readers from the other subjects (some of the Superior Achievers also showed isolated failures), but rather the
accumulation of deficits. As early as 1935, Castner (37) spoke

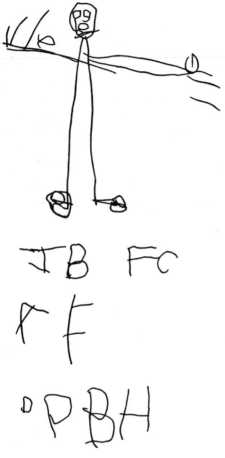

The boy whose work is shown above was of kindergarten age and average intelligence, but he was a Failing Reader by the end of the second grade. This very primitive figure was his attempt to draw a boy. The letters on the second and third lines are crudely copied, and he did not know their names. The bottom line shows his attempt to write his name, which is Martin. This representation has been reduced 70 per cent from the original.

of a *cluster* of traits which characterizes the kindergarten performance of children who tend to run into trouble with reading. Similarly, Hermann (105) emphasizes that the diagnosis of reading disability does not depend on any *single* pathognomonic sign, but on an appraisal of the whole configuration of dysfunctions.

We believe that such accumulation of deficits points to severe maturational lags, a concept advanced also by Bender (13), Cohn (43), and Subirana (222). Critchley (47) says ". . . most neurologists . . . would be reluctant to visualize in developmental dyslexia any focal brain lesion, dysplastic, traumatic, or otherwise. . . . To do so would be to ignore the important factors of immaturity as applied to chronological age, cortical development, and process of learning." Margaret Gutelius and Emma Layman

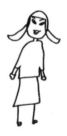

B F J C K A

NANCY

This is a sample of the work done by a girl of kindergarten age and average intelligence who was a Superior Achiever at the end of the second grade. When asked to draw a girl, she produced the above drawing. She was able to copy letters well and could write her own name. This representation has been reduced to 70 per cent from the original.

(88) go so far as to suggest discarding the term "specific reading disability" for the more general term "developmental lag."

OLDER CHILDREN WITH READING DIFFICULTIES

Clinical experience seems to show that these lags persist into later ages. The practical limitations of this study did not permit following the failing children beyond the second grade. As an alternate procedure, we inspected the records of older subjects—most of them boys, aged eleven to fifteen years—who had been referred to us in 1964 for severe reading, spelling, and writing difficulties. Those children who had been diagnosed by the referring psychiatrist or psychologist as primarily emotionally disturbed, as well as those whose history gave rise to a suspicion of brain injury, were not considered. The protocols of the sixteen remaining subjects were investigated. These older children came from middle to upper middle class homes; all of them attended private schools; their IQs ranged from 115 to 132.

Compared to the Failing Readers, these subjects—being older—were no longer hyperactive (32, 144). Their perceptuomotor lags seemed less severe. While Benton (17) maintains that such lags disappear entirely in older subjects, Silver and Hagin, (209), who followed severely retarded readers into young adulthood, reported persisting perceptuomotor deficits, and Bryant (29) found that most of his older reading disability cases continued to show minimal and subtle motor dysfunctions.

The over-all performance of these sixteen older children resembled in many ways that of the Failing Readers. The human-figure drawings of the older subjects were relatively crude and primitive, and their Bender Gestalten showed the lack of differentiation and the difficulties in synthesis and spatial organization that characterize a younger age group. Persisting deficits in all aspects of oral language were striking. Particularly prominent were short auditory-memory spans and diffuse auditory discrimination. Many of the older children showed word-finding difficulties, trouble with formulation and dysrhythmic, cluttered speech. Most of them were unable to tell a coherent story.

The handicaps of these older children in the graphomotor area were impressive: Many of them held the pencil the way beginners do and continued to struggle desperately with handwriting, which was jerky and messy and which usually broke down in compositions. A frequent association between poor handwriting and spelling difficulties has been reported in the literature (157, 176).

In our older group about half of the children had become fairly adequate readers; their intelligent use of contextual cues had enabled them to compensate for their early perceptual deficits. Bizarre spelling, as described by Roswell Gallagher (76), however, was a characteristic feature in this group. The children seemed to have continuing difficulties in maintaining a linguistic Gestalt (70); i.e., words looked different at different times and in different contexts (115, 122). Recall of printed configurations remained unstable.

Similar instability was observed at lower levels of CNS integration. These subjects showed for their age an unusually large number of concomitant movements (as observed on the finger-thumb-touching test); many of them had not yet established a functional superiority of one hand over the other. Identical phenomena have, of course, entirely different meanings at different ages. While concomitant movements and ambiguous lateralization are normal among young children, we feel that persisting associated movements, ill-defined lateralization, or deficits in right-left awareness in children over the age of eleven, if they occur in combination, reflect instability—Bender calls it plasticity—of CNS organization. Pervasive perceptuomotor instability, according to Bender (15), is the characteristic dysfunction in maturational lags.

In summary, the over-all performance of the older children, the so-called dyslexics,* seems to point to a profound and basic maturational deficit, a deficit so severe that one might speculate that it is rooted in the biological matrix, and constitutes a type of cerebral dysfunction.

In the older children investigated here, who came from a high social stratum and had superior intellectual endowment, this maturational deficit appeared to override intellectual, economic, and cultural determinants.†

When they were at kindergarten age, most of our older children must have functioned much like the Failing Readers. Whether *all* Failing Readers described here will continue to show massive difficulties, or whether a few, like the Slow Starters will "jell" at later ages, cannot be predicted from the data. On the basis of our clinical experience, however, we are prepared to say that unless the Failing Readers receive intensive remediation,‡ the gap between these children and their peers will become wider as the years go by, and that by the time they reach adolescence they will present multiple and perhaps irreversible handicaps. As the preceding pages show, these children display a characteristic configuration at preschool level that can be identified at early ages.

---

* Some educational psychologists object to the label "dyslexic"—largely for pragmatic reasons, because they believe it implies a "nihilistic" prognostic attitude. The heated dispute as to whether the dyslexic syndrome constitutes simply the extreme of the normal distribution in reading competence, or whether it is a distinctive syndrome, appears to be unproductive. Giants and dwarfs, for instance, are at the extremes of a bell-shaped curve, but show at the same time genuine endocrinological dysfunctions (personal communication, Dr. Maurice Charleton).

† While it is evident, as emphasized by Frank Riessman (193), that many poor readers belong to disadvantaged and minority groups, the study of the older children described here shows that severe physiological immaturity often outweighs socio-economic or ethnic factors.

‡ See Bryant's (30) recent paper on the remediation of severely disabled readers.

6
Prematurely Born Children

◆

The reader will recall that at the time the authors selected a group representative of the general population, they also chose a group of prematurely born children in order to evaluate the predictive effectiveness of the kindergarten tests for a *clinical* sample.

According to the definition accepted by the World Health Organization in 1948, a prematurely born child is one who weighs 2,500 grams (5 pounds, 8 ounces) or less at birth. Children whose birthweight falls below 2,500 grams, and who are by definition premature, do not constitute a homogeneous group. Cecil Drillien (60) mentions three categories: One consists of babies weighing less than five pounds, but born at term to mothers of small stature; another, of infants born at or near term but markedly underweight as a result of intrauterine malnutrition; the third, of children who are actually premature in terms of both weight and gestation time.

The clinical sample was selected from a group of 158 infants, born in 1955 and 1956, who had been cared for in the Premature Nursery of the Babies Hospital, Columbia-Presbyterian Medical Center, New York City, and had been investigated by Dr. William Silverman (210).

In the present study the exclusion criteria used in developing the general sample (see Chapter 2) were applied to the prematures and yielded a group of 53 prematurely born subjects whose birthweights ranged from 980 grams (2 pounds, 3 ounces) to 2,239 grams, (4 pounds, 15 ounces). In only six cases had gestation time been longer than thirty-seven weeks. At age three these children had been evaluated psychometrically and with regard to language development (129). Neurological examination had been done at the same time.

Although the two groups had been drawn from different populations, an evaluation of their background characteristics failed in most areas to reveal gross differences (see Appendix Table I-10). Age distributions were very similar. Slight differences in sex and race favored the prematurely born: This group contained more girls, who are thought to be more mature than boys of the same age (224) and more white children, who are believed to enjoy more cultural advantages than their Negro peers (53). The two groups were nearly identical with respect to mothers' employment outside the home, the number of times the children were read to each week, and kindergarten attendance.

On the other hand, among the prematures a significantly greater number of mothers had continued their own education beyond high school. (Hilda Knobloch and Benjamin Pasamanick (139), as well as Helen Wortis and Alfred Freedman (252), believe that the mother's educational status is a more reliable measure of environmental stimulation than is social status.) The two groups also differed as to IQ. The IQ levels of the prematurely born children were significantly lower than were those of the maturely born subjects, a fact that will be considered later. It is of interest in this context that Wortis and Freedman (252) found that the average IQ of prematurely born children of depressed socioeconomic status is lower than that of term children who live in the same deprived social environment.

PREDICTIONS FOR THE CLINICAL SAMPLE

In evaluating the predictive efficacy of the kindergarten tests for the prematurely born children, the same data collection procedures and correlation techniques used for the general population were applied (see Chapters 2 and 3).*

Appendix Table I-9 shows that a large number of perceptuo-motor and oral language tests administered at the kindergarten level predicted end-of-second-grade reading, writing, and spelling achievement not only for the general, but also for the clinical— the premature—group. Among the prematures, 22 kindergarten tests were significantly correlated with the ORP Index, 21 with spelling, and 22 with writing (as compared to 19, 20, and 16 tests, respectively, in the general sample). Many of the same kindergarten tests were significantly related to performance in *both* groups. However, there were differences. Predictors of later achievement were more numerous for the prematures than for the maturely born, particularly in the area of writing. Furthermore, in most cases the coefficient for the two groups differed in size, that for the prematures usually being the larger.

PERFORMANCE OF THE PREMATURELY BORN CHILDREN

The differences between the two groups were by no means confined to the area of prediction. We were struck above all by the fact that the prematures' maturational patterns seemed so much more erratic than that of the full-term children.

* The d_{yx} coefficient of correlation between each of the thirty-seven kindergarten tests and end-of-second-grade reading (ORP Index), spelling, and writing performance for both groups—prematurely and maturely born —are listed in Appendix Table I-9.

The literature on the subject of prematurity presents contra-dictory findings. Some writers (38, 138, 151), have maintained that, at kindergarten age, prematurely born children measure up to those born at term, provided that their IQs fall within the average range and that gross neurological sequelae are absent. A number of reports (16, 57, 60, 131), on the other hand, have commented on the high frequency of reading disabilities in pre-maturely born subjects. Helen Koch (141) speaks of possible ". . . subtle and long-time influences . . . of prematurity even in children who are accepted in normal school programs." Whether or not the deficits of prematurely born children persist into the early school years cannot, according to Gerald Wiener (249), be decided on the basis of studies done since 1940.

We had hoped that a careful investigation of the premature child's perceptuomotor, oral-language, and academic functioning might shed some light on the following questions: Is the perform-ance of prematurely born children at kindergarten age essentially different from that of children born at term? Do the prematurely and maturely born children progress at different rates during the developmentally crucial years between kindergarten and the end of second grade? Do the prematures at the end of their first and second grade in school read, write, and spell at the same level as their maturely born peers?

The chi-square test was used for two sets of comparisons:* (1) comparisons *within* the premature group according to sex and birthweight and (2) comparisons *between* the prematurely and the maturely born samples. These comparisons were based on that level of performance—called the "critical score level"—which yielded the best differentiation between the two groups tested.

---

* Yates' correction of the chi-square coefficient for small samples was employed where it was deemed appropriate.

THE FINDINGS

Comparisons Within the Premature Group

It was found that prematurely born *girls* perform better than prematurely born *boys* in reading, writing, and spelling at the end of both grades I and II. These differences reached statistically significant levels in writing and spelling at the end of second grade (see Appendix Table I-11). This confirms Sigrid Blegen's (24) findings as to the relatively poor performance of premature boys compared to premature girls and supports Wortis's and Freedman's (252) contention that males are particularly susceptible to the effects of prematurity.

Lightweight prematures have been reported to present greater hazards in learning than those whose weight approaches that of children born at term (60, 68, 93, 140). The findings relative to birthweight are reported here with reservations, because the prematurely born group in our study was, in effect, cut off at both extremes. There was only one child with a birthweight above 2,000 grams (4 pounds, 7 ounces) and only one with a birthweight below 1,000 grams (2 pounds, 3 ounces). Although this relative homogeneity would tend to reduce the relationship between weight and performance, the prematurely born children were nevertheless placed in three weight categories: 1,500 grams (3 pounds, 5 ounces) or less, 1,501 to 1,750 grams (3 pounds, 14 ounces), and 1,751 grams or more. Each weight group's performance in reading, writing, and spelling at the end of the first and second grade was then tabulated. No gradient in performance was found with ascending birthweight except in reading achievement at the end of the first grade. However, on four out of five scholastic tests children with birthweights below 1,500 grams performed less well than did subjects with higher birthweights (see Appendix Table I-12).

Comparisons Between Prematurely and Maturely Born Groups

The prematurely born children were then compared with the maturely born on each of the thirty-seven *kindergarten* tests. The most striking result was the almost uniformly poorer showing of the prematurely born subjects. The full-term children surpassed the prematures on 36 out of 37 performances; on 15 tests differences in favor of the maturely born children reached statistical significance. It is noteworthy that of these 15 tests, 11 were oral-language and reading readiness measures—in other words, performances that require a relatively high level of integrative competence.

As the data in Appendix Table I-14 show, on both the Over-all Reading Performance Index and the Writing Test at the end of Grade I the prematures did significantly less well than did the children born at term. At the end of Grade II, the prematures' performance in all three academic areas continued to be significantly inferior to that of maturely born subjects.

The possibility was next considered that the prematures, in spite of their poor showing on Grade II academic tests, might nevertheless, in the interval between kindergarten and the end of second grade, have shown signs of accelerated progress in some areas. This possibility was explored by readministering at the end of Grade II four kindergarten tests—Behavioral Control, Establishing of Hand Preference, Bender Visuo-Motor Gestalt Test, and Auditory Discrimination—and then determining whether the prematures had made greater progress in the intervening time, than had the children born at term. (The fact that the prematures had started at relatively low levels at kindergarten age and thus had clearly more room for improvement was taken into account in the statistical procedure.) The data show that except on the Bender Gestalt test, the prematurely born children had indeed progressed faster than the maturely born. (See Appendix Table I-15).

In *absolute* performance on the same tests, on the other hand, the term children continued to lead; only on the Bender Gestalt did the differences in favor of the maturely born children reach statistical significance (see Appendix Table I-16).

In summary, the prematurely born subjects functioned considerably less well than did the full-term children. While the former showed signs of "catching up" in some areas between the ages of five and a half and eight, their academic performance at the end of second grade continued to lag. While it is true that many of the prematurely born children had compensated for their original deficits, the findings in general are consistent with those of Lula Lubchenco and her associates (153), who report on the high incidence of academic failure and specific learning deficits among premature children of adequate intelligence.*

The findings were then reviewed in the light of three variables: intelligence, socio-economic background, and neurological status.

It will be remembered that the prematurely born children performed less well than did those born at term, not only on the kindergarten battery, but also on the Stanford-Binet Intelligence Test administered at the same time. However, the kindergarten tests and the Stanford-Binet, which is heavily loaded with verbal items, measure overlapping, although not identical, competences. It would therefore be inappropriate to try to account for group differences by Stanford-Binet scores. Because the competences evaluated by the two sets of tests do overlap, any attempt to "account" for IQ differences could be expected to reduce the observed disparity between groups.

It seemed of interest, nevertheless, to minimize the "effects" of intelligence by comparing the nineteen prematurely and the twenty-two maturely born subjects with IQs in the narrow range

* Clinical practice shows, however, that there are many prematurely born subjects with strong genetic endowment who perform at high levels.

between 90 and 105 on those fifteen kindergarten and academic tests which had originally discriminated significantly between groups. These comparisons showed the same trend reported previously—the prematurely born children did less well than the children who were born at term. On three tests—Concomitant Movements (related to CNS maturation), the Bender Visuo-Motor Gestalt Test (related to integrative competence), and end-of-second-grade reading—the differences attained statistical significance.

The socio-economic and educational status of the parents is widely regarded as being one of the determining factors in the reported differences between prematurely and maturely born children. Wiener (249) stresses the importance of controlling for social class in the investigation of prematurity. J. Douglas (58), in a British study of the mental ability and primary school progress of prematurely born subjects, found a number of striking handicaps, which were later shown to be of environmental origin. On the other hand, both Drillien (60) and Wortis and Freedman (252), who explored the relative contributions of prematurity and social environment, found that prematurely born children, many of whom show neurological deviations, are more vulnerable to the effects of an impoverished background than are children born at term—a finding that would suggest considerable interaction between the sociological and the physiological aspects of prematurity.

In our study, however, the educational achievement of the mothers in the prematurely born group was higher than that of the mothers of the maturely born. It seems highly unlikely, therefore, that socio-economic differences were determining factors in the poorer performance of our prematures. Gunborg Uddenberg's (232) findings were comparable. Although the mothers in his prematurely born sample came from the same social stratum as did the mothers of the control subjects, his prematurely born children did less well on perceptuomotor and reading tasks than did the subjects born at term. Similarly, Drillien (60), in her extensive study, found that prematurely born children are more likely to work at levels below their intellectual capacity than are full-term subjects of comparable intelligence and from similar homes.

The relatively poor performance of prematurely born children has often been ascribed to the higher frequency of brain injury in this group, the assumption being that interference with the integrity of the CNS would be reflected in widespread developmental and learning disturbances (27, 169). Harold Burks (31) suggests that reading disabilities may occur as sequelae of brain impairment and are related to difficulties in pattern making and physiological integration. In his hyperkinetic group there were five times as many prematurely born subjects as controls (32).

The limitations of the present project did not allow for neurological examination of the prematurely born children at the end of second grade. Thus, the effects of possible brain injury on academic achievement could not be *directly* assessed. It will be recalled, however, that records were available of the neurological evaluation of these subjects at the age of three; thus, we felt that it might be of interest to examine the prematurely born children's scholastic performance at age eight in the light of these early neurological findings.

Five of the forty-nine children examined at age three had been diagnosed as showing "definite or probable evidence* of neurological deficit." Of these five, three subjects passed and two failed reading and spelling tests at the end of second grade. It is possible that, among the three who passed, ongoing maturation had resolved most of the original problems; Charles Bradley (27) refers

---

* Squint, abnormal or extraneous ocular movements, hypotonia, motor retardation, deviating gait, seizures, and slow developmental history were considered to be manifestations of neurological dysfunction.

to a diminution in symptoms as children grow older. Since the number of our prematures with positive early neurological signs was so small, it was not possible to draw conclusions as to the relationship between positive neurological signs at early ages and subsequent learning difficulties.

On the other hand, of the forty-four children who at age three had shown no definite or probable neurological deficit,* twenty-three failed reading and spelling tests at age eight, perhaps because—as stressed by Thelander and his associates (228)—neurological examinations are not necessarily sensitive enough to pick up subtle dysfunctions. Thus, absence of *demonstrable* early neurological deficits in prematurely born children does not necessarily imply a good prognosis for learning at later ages. Subtle dysfunctions may persist (180) in aspects of the learning process which, like reading, writing, and spelling, require a high degree of differentiation and integration.

To ask whether the premature's inferior performance is related to actual neurological damage†—which interferes with the establishing of complex sensorimotor schemata—or to a severe and pervasive maturational lag, would fail to do justice to the complexity of the problem. The two may be related, since clinically, nonfocal brain injury may manifest itself primarily in disruption of or interference with crucial maturational processes (1).

CLINICAL IMPRESSIONS

Out of our continued contact with the prematurely born children—a contact that extended over a period of two and one-half years—have come some clinical observations.

* The term "minimal brain injury" has not been used here, since as Homer Reed (190) points out, the diagnosis is clearly inferential and criteria for it vary from one clinical setting to another.

† See the comprehensive and excellent paper by Wiener and his associates (250), which appeared after the conclusion of the present study.

We were struck by the diffuseness of these children and by their difficulty in mobilizing energy in the service of a goal. It is possible, of course, that maternal anxiety played a part here. David Kaplan and Edward Mason (127), as well as Thomas Oppé (174), have made the pertinent observation that the prematures' unusual appearance at birth, the prohibitions against the handling and fondling of these babies,* and their slow early development cannot but arouse profound anxiety in their mothers. Such maternal anxiety may flow over to the children and inhibit their freedom to function in a variety of ways. Maternal guilt, of course, may be another factor, since, the majority of prematurely born children are unwanted babies (23).

It seems likely, finally, that as a result of their early difficulties in homeostasis, motility, perceptuomotor patterning, and spatial orientation, prematurely born children are themselves more anxious and dependent than their full-term peers (11). Paul Schilder (201) believes that a child with disturbed equilibrium needs the help and support of his mother more than do others. It seems probable that prematurely born children pass through the normal stages of infantile dependency at a considerably later age than do children born at term. For instance, more "baby wishes" have been found among prematurely than among maturely born children (120). Such continuing dependency may be one other aspect of the prematures' physiological immaturity, which would make it difficult for them to become active participants in the learning situation.

Phyllis Greenacre (85) feels that the premature baby is predisposed to anxiety. In our sample the prematurely born subjects seemed much more vulnerable than the maturely born children.

---

* Such prohibitions may result in additional sensory deprivation, which in turn may contribute to relatively slow initial development. The question of whether prematurely born children are *able* to tolerate as much stimulation as full-term subjects has been dealt with by Oppé (174) and Koch (141).

Wortis and Freedman (252) believe that infants with defective or vulnerable nervous systems are especially sensitive to environmental pressures. Margaret Lawrence (149) speaks of injury to the ego apparatus as a result of physiological deficits. Perhaps it is because of such deficits that the ability of prematurely born children to tolerate stress of any kind seems to be low.

Clinically, the prematures appeared to be "different" from the children born at term. One of the authors, who had no knowledge of which subjects were prematurely born and which were not, had no difficulty identifying most of the prematurely born children. This identification was based as much on their general approach to work as on their test scores. The prematures' CNS functioning seemed more primitive, their behavioral controls less firmly established, their level of neurological integration lower than that of the maturely born. They presented subtle difficulties in motor, perceptual, visuomotor, and linguistic patterning—difficulties that extended into the early academic years and resulted in relatively inferior performance, especially with regard to tasks that required a high level of integration.

Thus, we found in our study that the prematurely born children did less well than the maturely born subjects on a large battery of tests administered at kindergarten age. While they showed some indications of "catching up" during the years between kindergarten and the end of second grade, significant lags persisted well into the eighth year of life. Prematurely born children, therefore, have to be regarded as an academic high-risk group. In view of the fact that at the very least 4 per cent (92) of school age youngsters in the United States are prematurely born, the findings reported here have more than theoretical relevance.

7

Maturational Lags

•

Both the Failing Readers, described in a previous chapter, and a large number of prematurely born subjects did poorly in reading at the end of the second grade. Our theoretical position, which is derived from clinical experience, is that difficulties with reading* are related to lags in neurophysiological maturation. In the following pages we re-examine this position in the light of the data collected in this study.

Maturation is the process of successive and overlapping changes in growth that take place in the physiological and psychological sectors of the organism. Development, according to Werner (246), proceeds from a state of relative globality and lack of differentiation in the direction of increasing articulation and hierarchic organization. The concept of maturation, as put forward by Bender (12), is based on the theory of functional areas in the brain and in the personality, which develop longitudinally according to a recognizable pattern. A maturational lag, then, would signify slow differentiation in this pattern. If successive stages of development represent levels of increasing complexity, then the perceptuomotor and linguistic performance of severely

* Only those reading and spelling difficulties are referred to here that are not related to psychiatric disturbance, brain injury, or extraneous factors such as frequent change of school, poor teaching, or deprived environmental conditions.

immature children—those who suffer from maturational lags—
can be expected to be less complex, less differentiated, and
more global than that of subjects whose development proceeds
smoothly.

The prematurely born children and the Failing Readers showed
behavior, motility, and finer motor coordination that was less well
patterned than that of their peers. Body image and visuomotor
experiences were primitive; the perceptual field was poorly structured and unstable; language reception was diffuse; expressive
tools were crude. In short, the two groups of children functioned
in ways characteristic of chronologically younger subjects.

In the case of the prematures it might be hypothesized that they
had started life with neurophysiological lags,* and that their
subsequent poor performance was related to the fact that they
had not altogether overcome these lags by the age of eight. In
the case of the Failing Readers, as in the children seen in clinical
practice, a genetically determined maturational defect (254)†
might have accounted for their poor showing. These are, of course,
conjectures. In any case, both the prematurely born children and
the Failing Readers failed a large number of tests administered
at kindergarten age.

That performance on these kindergarten tests reflects the children's maturational status and—if development is a consistent
process—that maturational status at early ages is *predictive* of
later functioning was our original assumption. This assumption

---

* Pasamanick and Knobloch (180) feel that the global reduction in intelligence of children with IQs below 80 reflects *gross* brain damage. The
insult to the organism in prematurely born children of *average* intelligence,
on the other hand, might be assumed to be diffuse rather than specific
and circumscribed, and to be reflected mainly in a disruption of the
maturational sequence.

† Unlike Orton (175) and a number of other researchers (90, 105, 119)
we believe, as do Zangwill (254) and Bender (13), that it is the *tendency
to immature patterning*, rather than the reading disability per se, which is
genetically determined.

was tested against the data on the basis of the following reasoning: Piaget (185) contends that the forming of complex or-
ganizations and schemes is an age-linked process. Gesell (80)
maintains that maturation is by and large a function of chronological age. If chronological age does, in fact, reflect maturational
level, then those kindergarten tests on which performance was
most closely related to chronological age should have been the
ones most sensitive to maturational differences. If, then, as we
believe, a child's maturational status at kindergarten age does
forecast his subsequent achievement, those tests that were most
sensitive to differences in maturation should have been the ones
that best *predicted* reading and spelling at the end of the second
grade.

On the basis of this reasoning, the kindergarten test were classified according to the degree to which each discriminated among
oldest, intermediate, and youngest kindergarten children.
This was done by determining the percentage of the oldest, the
intermediate, and the youngest subjects who obtained the critical
score level on a given test. Tests such as Word Recognition on
which the oldest children performed best, the intermediate subjects less well, and the youngest children worst, were characterized as "maturation-sensitive." Tests such as the Bender Gestalt,
on which the oldest children performed best and the youngest
performed worst, even though the intermediate group did not fall
clearly into line, were also considered to be maturation-sensitive,
though to a lesser degree. Those tests on which achievement was
not related to age were assumed not to be sensitive to maturational differences (see Appendix Table I-17).

Of the thirty-seven tests, fifteen differentiated among kindergarten children at three age levels; ten discriminated between the
oldest and youngest subjects; and twelve tests failed to reveal
differences. Of the thirty-seven tests, twenty-five, thus, could be
described as maturation-sensitive.

The expectation that the maturation-sensitive tests would predict later achievement better than the "nonmaturation-sensitive" tests was borne out by the findings. Of the maturation-sensitive tests, 76 per cent were significantly correlated with second-grade achievement, compared to only 17 per cent of the nonmaturation-sensitive tests (see Appendix Table I-18).

Piaget's (185) and Gesell's (79) assumption that chronological age reflects maturation is true for the majority of children. Chronological age is a fairly workable predictor of subsequent performance. (As shown in a previous chapter, chronological age was significantly related to later achievement, though the coefficient was low.) The focus of this study, however, was on those children of adequate intelligence in whom chronological age does *not* reflect developmental level, the children who suffer from maturational lags and who therefore present a high risk of academic failure. For these children chronological age alone is not only inadequate, but misleading as a predictor. There were eighteen children in this study who were over six and a half years old at the time of first-grade entrance. On the basis of chronological age, these children should have succeeded, but four of them failed in reading and spelling at the end of the second grade.

The maturation-sensitive tests administered at kindergarten level, on the other hand, identified as potential failures three of these four older children. (Data for the fourth were incomplete.) This supports our contention that maturational status is actually the crucial factor in forecasting subsequent achievement.

In summary, these findings, as well as clinical experience, support our position that there is indeed a close link between a child's maturational status at kindergarten age and his reading and spelling achievement several years later.

8
Some Clinical Observations

＊

STYLE OF APPROACH

The design of our study provided for several contacts with the fifty-three project children in the general sample over a period of two and a half years. It thus afforded an opportunity to observe some facets of the children's behavior which, although they did not bear directly on the investigation's chief aim of prediction, may nevertheless be of interest.

One set of observations was concerned with the way in which the children met the testing situation—in other words, with their approach to learning and their characteristic style of functioning. Consideration was also given to the question of consistency of style over the next two and a half years and its relative significance in terms of academic performance. (No attempt was made to relate style of functioning to underlying dynamics.)

The assessment of the children's approach to the testing situation was based on notes in the chart and on the profile written about each youngster after the initial kindergarten session. A review of these notes and profiles showed that the children could be grouped, roughly, into four different categories, according to their particular style of functioning.

Group I consisted of twelve subjects who, despite some mild anxiety early in the session, were remarkably self-confident and clearly "on top of" the situation, in the sense that they participated actively and responsibly in what was going on, and seemed to organize themselves and their environment without apparent effort. They worked independently and appeared to channel all of their considerable "organismic energy" toward the tasks presented.* Most of these five- and six-year olds asked pertinent questions, and were delighted when they arrived at what seemed to be the appropriate solutions to a problem. At the same time, they were able to look at their own performance critically and objectively. Since the material itself exerted considerable pull, these children were able to work without prodding; their enjoyment of mastery for its own sake pointed to a measure of ego autonomy. At the end of the initial kindergarten session, most of them expressed a desire to come back.

Few changes in style of functioning were observed in this particular group over the next thirty-two months. One boy, who had seemed rather anxious at the end of his first year at school, was his old, confident self again when seen at the end of the second grade; another boy—the only one in this group who had seemed to be somewhat involved in fantasies in kindergarten—appeared to have "emerged" by the age of eight.

As might have been expected, the performance of these twelve children in Group I, both at kindergarten and subsequently at elementary school age, was most satisfactory. It seems likely that their early confident and mature approach to work reflected the same advanced state of ego organization as did their later superior achievement.

Group II consisted of twenty-one subjects who were as effective academically as the children in Group I, but whose style of functioning was totally different. These children, unlike those in Group I, did not seem to enjoy the challenge provided by the tests.

* See White (248) and also the discussion of Escalona and Heider (64) on "availability" of energy.

Their anxiety and tension were marked. They made frequent trips to the bathroom. Although most of these children lacked self-confidence, they were conscientious, driving, and very ambitious. While they were clearly concerned over performance, they did not seem to be motivated by the rewards inherent in mastery for its own sake, but instead by a need for recognition and approval from the adult. They were not, however, immobilized by their anxiety, their fear of failing, and their difficulties with decisions, but were able to marshal their energy in the service of the goal; in fact, their meticulous and somewhat obsessive approach appeared to be, if anything, an asset in terms of performance at this early level.* These children functioned well, although clearly at some cost to themselves.

Nine of the twenty-one subjects in Group II showed evidence of a change in style over the following two and a half years. One boy, who had seemed almost entirely paralyzed at the end of the first grade, as a result of excessive parental pressure (which was subsequently reduced), appeared to be freer at the end of the second grade. Another child seemed to be less inhibited; a third, less fantasy-ridden. In general, changes were consistently in the direction of decreased anxiety and increased self-confidence.

To our surprise, two children in Group II achieved high scores on second-grade tests despite major upheavals at home—in one case a mother's, in the other a father's nervous breakdown. For these two youngsters, the academic area must have been relatively conflict-free—in fact, they may well have found in the school setting a source of satisfaction and support.

The compliant and well-behaved children in Group II were, of course, destined to become popular with their teachers, and it is quite possible that their academic success and their popularity with those in authority resulted in reduction of anxiety and increase in self-confidence as well as in a more positive self image.

---

* We doubt that the same anxious approach would be equally effective in the higher grades in school.

The eight children in Group III again were very different: They were boisterous, cheerful, and happy-go-lucky, but their difficulties with behavioral control were severe. Four of them showed evidence of disorganization, of hyperactivity, distractibility, and disinhibition. While they were clearly delighted with the attention they received and with the candy abundantly provided for them, they were on the whole not interested in the tests themselves. They had not yet learned, as Anna Freud (71) describes it, ". . . to carry out preconceived plans with a minimum regard for the lack of immediate pleasure yield, intervening frustration, and a maximum regard for the pleasure in the ultimate outcome. . . ." These children, like chronologically younger subjects, were unable to maintain the tension required for tasks that did not provide immediate gratification. Although these vigorous and vivid youngsters seemed to have abundant "organismic energy," they were unable to mobilize this energy in a goal-directed way. We felt that this inability was but one aspect of their pervasive organismic immaturity, which was reflected in physiological as well as in psychological aspects of functioning consistent with the observations of Heinz Hartmann and his co-workers (99), namely, that there is an interaction between maturation and the formation of psychic structure. Lucille Barber (7) believes that "immature" ego development in certain children is part of their over-all maturational lag.

As might have been suspected, most of the children in Group III did poorly on practically all kindergarten tests.

By the time two years had elapsed, one boy in this group had learned to focus and to apply himself. Another had changed from a seemingly cheerful, unconcerned youngster to one so preoccupied with performance—he was doing well at the time—that the pediatrician was afraid "he would develop ulcers." (We were unable to account for this change, since an interview with the mother threw little light on the dynamics of the boy's disturbance.) Of the six remaining children in this group, three passed

reading tests at the end of the second grade; three others, however, belonged to the group of Failing Readers described in a
previous section.

Group IV consisted of eleven children who found the testing
extremely burdensome. Most of them seemed bewildered and
overwhelmed, and had difficulties in getting oriented. As do the
children described in a recent paper by L. F. Kurlander and
Dorothy Colodny,* they had trouble organizing their internal
and external world. These children were anxious, but their
anxiety was amorphous and diffuse, in contrast to that of the
subjects in Group II, whose anxiety was focused on performance.
The children in Group IV were passive, infantile, and dependent
youngsters; almost all of them had to be dragged through the
long initial kindergarten examination. Problems with behavioral
control were evident in about half of them. Ego strength in seven
of the eleven subjects seemed to be poor. At the time of the
kindergarten testing, only nine of the fifty-three children from the
general sample had received a below-average rating on ego
strength. Seven of the nine children so rated belonged to the
group under discussion here.

Among these passive and dependent children, some showed
more or less subtle changes over the next thirty-two months. One
boy, who had had a good year in first grade, reverted to his
kindergarten pattern during the second grade; the remaining
children, however, became somewhat less dependent and less
infantile. One changed from a passively angry child into one who
was overtly angry. Another, though still slightly deviating, had
learned to handle himself more effectively and now presented a
more conventional facade. In spite of these changes, seven of the
eleven children in this group continued to perform poorly at the

---

* See L. F. Kurlander and Dorothy Colodny, " 'Pseudoneurosis' in the
Neurologically Handicapped Child," *American Journal of Orthopsychiatry*,
35 (1965), 733–738.

end of the second grade—in fact, all but one of them were classified as Failing Readers.

While at least four different styles of approach could thus be identified at early ages, style was not necessarily related to later achievement. Both the self-confident (Group I) and the tense and anxious (Group II) subjects performed at high levels on academic tasks. Diametrically opposed findings are reported as to the significance of anxiety for learning. One study (200) states that anxiety level in high-ability seventh graders is positively related to language arts. On the other hand, E. Duwayne Keller and Vinton Rowley (132) conclude that anxiety scores have a negative correlation with both intelligence and school achievement.

In the group investigated here, a modicum of disturbance was apparently not necessarily detrimental to success. One boy might serve as an example: He did well academically, in spite of the fact that he vomited each morning before going to kindergarten and appeared at the end of the second grade with a bald spot, the result of compulsive hair-pulling. Children respond differently to emotional stress: The degree to which academic functioning is affected by emotional conflict varies from child to child; it depends also on the nature and intensity of the conflict. The relationship between psychological disturbance and school performance is clearly complex and by no means easy to assess.

What struck us was the consistency of the subjects' approach to learning and the inherent continuity of behavioral style.* The majority of children investigated here—at least two-thirds of them—were very much the same kind of youngsters at the end of the second grade as they had been at kindergarten age; the assertive child remained assertive, the tense child continued to be tense. Changes seemed to be in keeping with earlier behavior and were, for the most part, in the direction of better ability to

---

* This consistency is beautifully illustrated in the book by Escalona and Heider (64).

cope. These changes may thus be regarded as a function of ongoing development in the broadest sense.

MODALITY STRENGTH AND WEAKNESS

A second set of observations dealt with relative strength and weakness in the auditory and visual modalities at kindergarten age. In some children, information is absorbed more easily through auditory pathways; in others, learning is facilitated primarily by using visual channels. Werner and Bernard Kaplan (247) refer to individual differences in pace and direction of development in the different perceptual areas. Wepman (245) has explored differential rates of maturation in the various modalities. In our study, relative strength in the visual- and auditory-perceptual areas was investigated by comparing the children's performance on four tests in the realm of *auditory*-perceptual organization (Imitation of Tapped Patterns, Auditory Discrimination, Language Comprehension, and the Gates Rhyming Test) with their performance on four tests involving *visual*-perceptual competence (Bender Visuo-Motor Gestalt, Horst, Gates Matching, and Word Recognition tests).

When the children's performance on these two sets of tests was compared, few if any differences were found between auditory- and visual-perceptual ability in 43 of the 53 subjects. This was true along the whole range of performance from excellent to poor. The superior visualizers performed at a high level on auditory-perceptual tests, while the inferior visualizers did poorly with auditory-perceptual tasks.* To all intents and purposes then,

---

* Birch and Belmont (21), in a highly ingenious experiment, explored intermodal equivalence; the child's ability to integrate intersensory—that is to say, auditory and visual—information. They found that the capacity to make such equivalence judgments was positively correlated with reading test scores in first and second grades, and suggested that this competence is crucial for the acquisition of reading skills. Only 30 per cent of the

43 out of 53 subjects showed no modality preference, and the organism's level of integrative competence seemed to be reflected in both the auditory and the visual realms.

Discrepant modality patterning at kindergarten age, however, was found in ten subjects—that is, 19 per cent of the children were markedly superior in one modality as compared to the other. Of these ten children, seven did very well auditorily but showed striking deficits in the visual-perceptual area. Three children presented the opposite picture: While they failed all auditory-perceptual tests, they excelled in visual-perceptual ones.

Varying interpretations have been offered for such striking modality discrepancies. Psycho-analytically oriented observers, such as Victor Rosen (195), feel that modality preference is related to early libidinal cathexis; other researchers have found modality-bound deficits in cases of minimal or gross brain injury. Jean Martin Charcot, as reported by Sigmund Freud (72) in 1891, interpreted modality preference in terms of the individual's inherent endowment. As early as 1883, Sir Francis Galton (74) discussed differences in "imagery types." Escalona and Heider (64) were impressed with infants' varying responses to stimulation in the different modalities.

When we reviewed the academic performance of the ten children who at kindergarten age had demonstrated discrepant modality patterning,* we found the following:

---

kindergarten children tested by Birch, however, were capable of integrating auditory with visual information at better than chance levels. One would hazard the guess that the superior visualizers and auditors in the present kindergarten sample would fall into this category.

* It would have been preferable to retest modality preference at the end of the second grade. We felt, however, that the data available—two retests in the auditory and only one in the visual realm—were not sufficient to permit even tentative conclusions on this basis. Escalona and Heider (64) found changes in modality sensitivity between infancy and age five. Thus, it is possible that changes in modality preference may also have occurred in our sample in the interval between ages five and eight.

The three children who had been superior visualizers at kindergarten age received high scores on end-of-second-grade reading tests. This might have been expected in view of the fact that visual determinants are far more crucial in the reading process than are auditory ones (94). In a number of children, there appears to be a direct road from the printed representation of the word to its meaning. Such children apparently do not need the auditory and kinesthetic image of the word; like the highly skilled readers discussed by Friedrich Kainz (126), they seem to proceed directly from the printed symbol to the underlying concept. Children with marked visual-perceptual deficits, on the other hand, have to translate—vocally or subvocally—a sequence of letters seen into a sequence of sounds heard, and it is these auditory sequences, not the printed configurations, that in turn release meaning (113).

Of the seven subjects who were gifted auditorily but were poor visualizers, five passed and two failed all reading tests at the end of the second grade. These five auditorily gifted children who read well had been intensively trained in phonics, according to reports obtained from teachers,* and were thus able to utilize their auditory competence to compensate for deficits in visual-perceptual ability. They might have failed had they been exposed exclusively to the sight method; in fact, the two poor visualizers who failed all reading tests had not received phonic training.

We feel that exploration of modality strength and weakness is of more than theoretical interest and should largely determine teaching methods.† Children who do well in both auditory and visual modalities will benefit from either sight or phonic techniques, but they will presumably do best with a combination.

---

* Information as to teaching methods used in each child's classroom was collected for all project children.

† A differential diagnosis of perceptual and linguistic assets and deficits, useful for remediation, is provided by the Illinois Test of Psycholinguistic Ability (137).

Children who perform poorly in both modalities are in need of a multiple approach; they require, in fact, activation of as many learning pathways as possible, including kinesthetic and motor ones (66). Youngsters who have severe visual-perceptual deficits but who are good auditors require heavy emphasis on phonics, which will enable them to compensate for their shortcomings in the visual realm by means of their auditory competence.

In our opinion, therefore, one method of teaching cannot be favored over another as a matter of principle. (Most discussions of the subject seem to miss this point.) Approaches to teaching should depend on the individual child's strengths and weaknesses in the different modalities.

9
Recommendations

●

Whatever the theoretical orientation, it is generally acknowledged that crucial changes in both the physiological and psychological sectors of the organism take place in the period between five-and-a-half and eight years, the time considered in our investigation. Theta frequencies (147)° and the whirling response largely disappear (15); important qualitative changes occur in cognition (186); secondary processes emerge upon resolution of the Oedipal conflict (182).°

It is thus hazardous at best to predict performance and behavior from data collected at a time when the organism is still so very much in flux. Nevertheless, our findings suggest that it is possible to predict end-of-second-grade achievement on the basis of kindergarten functioning. We therefore recommend that a predictive index of the kind described in Chapter 4 be administered to all children during the second half of their kindergarten year, and that the decision as to first-grade entrance be based by and large on the child's score on this index.

The index is, of course, only a formula, and it would be unfortunate if it were to draw the teacher's attention away from

° Theta frequencies are brain waves of five to seven cycles per second. The whirling response is the tendency of the body to follow the head when it is being turned to the right or left. Secondary processes refer to ego activities which are no longer under the dominance of unconscious drives.

the child's actual performance and behavior. Rather than being a substitute for observation, the index should assist the teacher in translating her often excellent but sometimes impressionistic judgment of the child's readiness into a more specific assessment of his perceptuomotor and linguistic functioning.

"Readiness" is a controversial subject. However, it seems clear that no real dichotomy exists between readiness conceived of as an intrinsic state of the organism, and readiness viewed primarily as the result of stimulation and teaching (9). Maturation, as interpreted by Piaget (185), Kurt Koffka (142), and Donald Hebb (101) is contingent on functioning—which, in turn, is fostered by experience and training. Schilder (201) feels that training plays a significant part even in those functions in which maturation of the CNS is of primary importance. Maturation unfolds in continuous interaction with stimulation. Thus, the educator cannot afford to wait passively for maturation to occur, as was done in the 1920s, nor should he expose the child to a kind of instruction that is clearly inappropriate at his particular stage of growth. What is desirable is to match teaching methods to the child's specific developmental needs.

What does a match between developmental level and instruction mean, in terms of the children who have been identified by the Predictive Index as high risks? In our educational system, entrance into first grade is based solely on chronological age. As has been discussed in a preceding chapter, however, chronological age is not always a reliable indicator of a child's readiness. Hale Shirley (205) estimates that 15 per cent of the children reaching school age are not ready for reading instruction, as the result of the single factor of immaturity. Ilg and Ames (118) put the proportion of "overplaced" children much higher—at approximately 50 per cent—in an upper middle class community.

To admit very immature youngsters into first grade, where their chances to succeed are slim, and where, at the very beginning of their school careers, they are exposed to the damaging experience of failure, is highly undesirable. The psychological stresses experienced by children who are not ready for the educational demands of first grade have been described by Jack Novick (172). Allowing "non-ready" children to enter first grade, in the belief that they will "outgrow" their difficulties, is a procedure fraught with hazards. Immature first graders do not necessarily "catch up," but instead they tend to fall further behind (18, 118).

We suggest, therefore, that the schools institute small "transition classes" between kindergarten and first grade for children who, regardless of age, are not "ready." Such "maturity classes" have been introduced in Norway and Sweden, in spite of the fact that first-grade entrance there is set at age seven (223).

Immature children's developmental timing is atypical. At kindergarten age they are unable to benefit from prereading programs. Repeating kindergarten would give them an additional year to mature in and might thus have certain advantages, but it would not provide the intensive and specific training these children need. Promotion into first grade, on the other hand, would not solve their problem either, since the pace in first grade is usually too fast for those youngsters who are ready to learn, but are as yet unable to cope with organized reading and writing instruction at the conventional age.

The transition class, on the other hand, would start on the ground floor. It would aim at stabilizing the child's perceptuo-motor world and would take him—in slow motion, as it were—through a program in which each step is carefully planned. This class would carry him to the point where he would be able to benefit from formal education. Teaching methods in such a class, unlike those in first grade, which provide more or less uniform training for all children, would be tailored to the pupil's individual needs.

The transition class would be considerably more structured than are kindergarten groups and would help the immature and "scattered" child to function, first on a relatively simple and later on a more complex plane. The transition class would be small, enabling the teacher to give massive support to the anxious and dependent youngster who tends to be overwhelmed in a setting which does not provide individual guidance. [Reduction of class size for the least able pupils is strongly recommended by the Philadelphia Improvement Program (124).]

Needless to say, the teacher in such a transition class would have to have special qualifications, since, in addition to structure and careful organization, immature children require a greater than usual degree of tolerance and empathy.

A variety of problems could be dealt with in the transition class.° Seating the hyperactive youngster close to the teacher would protect him from the barrage of environmental stimuli. Activities like hopping, skipping, ball bouncing, and throwing would provide gross motor outlets for those children who are as yet unable to sit still for extended periods, and would, at the same time, foster large motor patterning (135, 198).

The transition class would assist the disoriented child who has trouble with patterning of time and space, who seems to be walking around in a fog, who does not really know what is happening in the classroom, who has little awareness of *when* important events will take place, or *where* they will occur. This sort of youngster looks lost and bewildered; much of his energy seems to be taken up by attempts to find his bearings; thus, little is available for learning.

Teaching this type of child the layout of the school, the position of the classroom, the direction in which his home lies is often helpful in a general way. Basically, however, orientation in *space* starts with the development of a cohesive body image. The child's awareness of his own body, its parts, and their relationship to

° A wealth of suggestions is offered in the book on teaching methods for brain-injured and hyper-active children by William Cruickshank and his associates (48). Many of their suggestions apply not only to brain-injured subjects, but also to the immature.

each other is essential for establishing left-right discrimination and consistent left-to-right progression. Thus, help with the development of a cohesive body image would be part of the teaching program.

To become oriented in *time*, the child would participate in the planning of his daily schedule. He would be taught the changes in the seasons and the time of school opening and closing. To grasp temporal relationships is often surprisingly difficult for immature children, and they may need very concrete clues so as to remember sequences such as the days of the week. Any sequence represents an organization in time, and learning to perceive, to process, to store, and to recall the serial order of information is a requisite for later reading activities. Training in this area must, however, start on a nonverbal level. Mary Masland (161) suggests tapping out rhythmic patterns on the child's own body. Rhythmic experiences such as marching and swinging to music are helpful.

Difficulties with *verbal communication* are a central problem in youngsters with maturational lags; many of them neither listen nor talk. Verbal give and take is fostered by the teacher who directs himself to the child's basic and immediate needs. Communication has both receptive and expressive aspects. On the receptive side, ability to listen cannot be taken for granted. Some children continue to be dependent on movement as a means of coming to terms with the world around them, and fail to attend to the spoken word. Their short auditory memory spans and their undifferentiated auditory discrimination, moreover, interfere with interpretation of what they hear. Auditory discrimination practice clarifies auditory-perceptual Gestalten for the child whose language reception is diffuse; it is an essential aspect of training in a transition class. The verbal output of immature and deprived children* usually reflects their diffuse reception. Defective articulation, primitive sentence construction, immature syntax,

---

* Many culturally deprived children are physiologically immature. Evidence by June Fite and Louise Schwartz (67) seems to show that con-

often massive word-finding difficulties, awkward formulations, all constitute a severe handicap often long beyond the elementary grades. The teacher in the transition class helps the child first and foremost to use words as the preferred form of communication. Learning to express feelings and experiences verbally precedes instruction in the more formal features of communication. Only at a later stage would the child get assistance with articulatory patterning and with syntactical forms.

Communicative difficulties are often complicated by *conceptual* deficits. Many five and six year olds do not comprehend the small, abstract words and phrases such as "on top of," "before," or "because," which represent spatial, temporal, and causal relationships. Failure to grasp the meaning of words such as "same" and "different" may interfere with the child's performance on reading readiness tasks which require him to discriminate between "same" and "different" configurations. Conceptual training, therefore, as stressed by Deutsch (55), belongs in a prereading curriculum.

That children with reading disorders have trouble with *visual* perception is common knowledge. Their perception may be fragmented; they may be unable to organize discrete clues into meaningful wholes. The question is: At what level of visual perception do they encounter difficulties? Visual perception is not a unitary process. There is, on the simplest plane, the differentiation between the familiar and the unfamiliar; to distinguish an object from its mirror image is more difficult. Identification of and discrimination between "critical" features of letter configurations is at the heart of most reading readiness programs. The immature child, however, must start with a more basic experience, with figure-ground discrimination. Teaching the child to pull out the relevant figure from a strongly structured ground promotes the organization of the visual field. The use of clay

---

stitutional deficits are more frequent in disadvantaged populations than in others and that in such groups emotional and social factors compound the original difficulties. See also M. Deutsch (55) and William Sheldon (203).

and sand for setting off a variety of forms embedded in a neutral ground provides a combination of visual and kinesthetic figure-ground experiences. Research in Russia (255) has shown that small children are better able to understand the relationship between parts of objects when they manipulate these objects. Visual analysis is facilitated by a combination of manipulation and visual exploration. The handling of plastic or plywood letters assists the children to make the subtle discriminations required for the recognition of individual letter shapes. Tracing, stenciling, and copying letters serves to integrate the visual with the graphic Gestalt of the word.

Immature children do not necessarily understand the fact that letters seen represent sounds heard. Before teaching them the sound equivalents of letters, one must make sure that they grasp the basic principles involved. The next step, the blending of sounds into words, is an exacting process and can be undertaken only when the child is ready for the analysis and synthesis required.

Prolonged and intensive prereading training in a transition class would, finally, provide an opportunity to translate into educational practice the insights gained from a careful scrutiny of the child's weakness and strength in the various modalities as revealed by the Predictive Index. A transition class would permit the exploration of each child's assets and deficits in the auditory and visual areas, as discussed in Chapter 8. Instruction would be geared differentially to children with auditory-perceptual difficulties and to those with gaps in visual perception. During certain times of the day youngsters with receptive- and expressive-language deficits would receive specific language training. Others would get assistance with visual discrimination and configurational techniques. A third group would work on directional and graphomotor patterning. In short, the transition class would serve to help children to fill in specific gaps in some areas and to utilize their assets in others.

Marie van Hoosan (234) has called the interval between kindergarten and first grade the "twilight zone" of learning. It is this twilight period which is served by the transition class.

A few children in such a class would be integrated into the regular first grade after a few weeks or months of intensive training. Most others would be ready to cope with first grade a year later. Carleton Washburne (237) reports that by the end of the third grade, those pupils who had started reading instruction later than others had caught up with their peers; by the end of the eighth grade, they were a year and a half ahead.* A small number of children suffering from severe and persisting lags might require continuing help for at least two or three years. Beth Slingerland (214) describes a program of prevention for young children presenting specific language disabilities. Those of her first graders who do poorly on nonstandardized tests receive instruction in separate classes and, in severe cases, are retained there up to five and six years.

At present, most school systems do not provide remedial help for children who fail in reading and spelling until the end of the third grade. This is unfortunate because the development of perceptual and language functions probably follows a sequence analogous to that in organic, morphological development (43). Deutsch (52) speaks of "critical" periods in cognitive growth; Mildred McGraw's (158) work demonstrates that there are specific times in the child's life when the organism is especially susceptible to certain kinds of stimulation. The basic perceptuomotor functions that underlie reading may be harder to train at the end of the third grade than they are earlier, during "critical" developmental stages. By the end of the third grade, moreover, emotional problems and phobic responses resulting from continued

---

* In a very recent research project Spache, *et al.*, show that an intensified and extended reading readiness program has beneficial effects on reading achievement, in spite of the delay in introducing formal reading. (See George Spache, *et al.*, "A Longitudinal First Grade Reading Program," 19 (1966), 580–584.)

failure may have so complicated the original difficulties that they may no longer be reversible.

The early identification of high-risk children was the goal of our investigation. Identification, however, is only a first step toward reversing a situation that now results in an unjustifiable waste of educational opportunities. A second step is equally essential: High-risk children must be provided at the earliest possible time with an educational approach that will enable them to realize their potential and to become productive members of the community.

A FINAL WORD

Twenty years of clinical experience with intelligent, but educationally disabled children, whose learning drive has become severely damaged, has convinced us that many of these children would not have required help had their difficulties been recognized at early ages. Early identification would have obviated the need for later remedial measures.

This study has attempted to develop techniques for the early identification of children who, at kindergarten age, seemed to present a specific pattern of dysfunctions, reflecting an underlying developmental lag.

Children's developmental rhythm varies widely. Recognition of and respect for these variations are crucial at a time when society places increased pressures for early achievement on both children and parents. Such recognition implies the taking of active educational measures geared to the child's individual needs at his particular developmental level.

The great Swiss educator Johannes Pestalozzi (183) said in 1802, "Thus to instruct men is nothing more than to help human nature to develop in its own way, and the art of instruction depends primarily on harmonizing our messages and the demands we make upon the child with his powers at the moment."

Appendix I

Tables

—

Table I-1. Grade II Over-all Reading Performance Index Scores[a]
(for children in the general sample)

ORP Index Score	Number	Gates Advanced Primary Score (grade)	Gray Oral Score (grade)
Advanced reader	16	3.5 or above	3.5 or above
Better than adequate reader	12	3.5 or above	2.5–3.4
	2	2.5–3.4	3.5 or above
Adequate reader	10	2.5–3.4	2.5–3.4
	2	3.5 or above	2.4 or below
Less than adequate reader	5	2.5–3.4	2.4 or below
	1	2.4 or below	2.5–3.4
Poor reader	5	2.4 or below	2.4 or below

[a] ORP Index scores are in terms of Gray and Gates Reading Test scores.

Table I-2. D_{yx} Coefficients of Correlation Between 37 Kindergarten Tests
and Grade II Achievement Tests
(for children in the general sample)

| Kindergarten Test | Grade II Test | | |
	ORP Index	Writing	Spelling
Behavioral patterning: Hyperactivity, Distractibility and Disinhibition Index	.46*	.48†	.40*
Motility patterning: Concomitant Movements	.03	.05	.04
Gross motor patterning:			
Balance	.09	—.15	.14
Hopping	.22	.18	.18
Throwing	.10	.06	.14
Fine motor patterning:			
Pegboard Speed Index	.17	.27*	.23*
Tying a Knot	.13	.38	—.16
Pencil Use	.34*	.46†	.27
Body image: Human-figure Drawing	.23*	.11	.20*
Laterality: Hand Preference Index	.10	.18	.15
Visual-perceptual patterning:			
Figure-ground Organization	.05	.16	.12
Bender Visuo-Motor Gestalt	.44†	.33†	.45†
Auditory-perceptual patterning:			
Tapped Patterns	.30*	.23	.36*
Auditory Memory Span	.28	.29	.20
Auditory Discrimination (Wepman)	.26*	.11	.31*
Word Recognition (Peabody)	.21	.16	.26*
Language Comprehension	.21	.06	.20
Expressive language:			
Consonant Articulation	.12	.01	.03
Articulatory Stability	.16	—.17	.24
Word Finding	.20	.18	.26
Story Organization	.28*	.05	.27*
Number of Words	.40†	.27*	.32*
Sentence Elaboration	.18	.16	.23
Number of Grammatical Errors	.09	.01	.07
Definitions (Binet)	.07	.14	.10
Categories	.24*	.23*	.36*
Reading readiness:			
Name Writing	.43†	.30*	.32*
Copying of Letters	.16	.35*	.30*

Kindergarten Test	Grade II Test		
	ORP Index	Writing	Spelling
Letter Naming	.55†	.34*	.56†
Reversals (Horst)	.36†	.25†	.34*
Word Matching (Gates)	.35†	.19*	.37*
Word Rhyming (Gates)	.22*	.13	.15
Word Recognition I (Pack)	.40†	.38†	.39†
Word Recognition II (Table)	.48†	.24*	.45†
Word Reproduction	.42†	.31†	.39†
Style:			
Ego Strength	.48*	.35*	.39*
Work Attitude	.43*	.38*	.46†

* .01 ≤ P ≤ .05.
† P ≤ .01.

Table I-3. D_{yx} Coefficients of Correlation Between Selected Items of Background Information and Grade II Achievement Tests (for children in the general sample)

Background Information	Grade II Test		
	ORP Index	Writing	Spelling
Family history			
Oral language difficulties	—.17	.09	—.19
Reading-spelling difficulties	.17	.04	.12
Left-handedness or ambidexterity	.11	.03	.05
Verbal stimulation			
Ordinal position	.02		
Mother's education	.19		
Mother's employment status	.22		
Exposure to story telling	.01	—.09	.02
Child's response to reading	.03	.05	.05
Child's response to TV	.20	.04	.15
Kindergarten attendance	.07	.00	.05
IQ	.31*	.05	.19
Chronological age (Grade I entrance)	.23		

* .01 ≤ P ≤ .05.

Table I-4. D_{yx} Coefficients of Correlation Between Grade II ORP Index and Potentially Predictive Kindergarten Tests,[a] by IQ
(for children in the general sample)

Test	All Children (N = 53)	IQ 106 or Below (N = 26)	IQ 107 or Above (N = 27)
Hyperactivity, Distractibility, and Disinhibition Index	.46	.61	.21
Pencil Use	.34	.30	.29
Human-figure Drawing	.23	.39	—.21
Bender Visuo-Motor Gestalt	.44	.55	.34
Tapped Patterns	.30	.16	.35
Auditory Discrimination (Wepman)	.26	.29	.14
Story Organization	.28	.46	.13
Number of Words	.40	.55	.04
Categories	.24	.23	.22
Name Writing	.43	.40	.17
Letter Naming	.55	.34	.37
Reversals (Horst)	.36	.27	.33
Word Matching (Gates)	.35	.19	.44
Word Rhyming (Gates)	.22	.15	.25
Word Recognition I (Pack)	.40	.29	.47
Word Recognition II (Table)	.48	.28	.63
Word Reproduction	.42	.39	.33
Ego Strength	.48	.47	.29
Work Attitude	.43	.44	.30

[a] Since the distribution of the data did not permit the use of multiple and partial regression techniques to control for intelligence, an alternate method was employed. The total group was divided into two subgroups according to IQ, and separate coefficients of correlation were computed for the kindergarten tests that had been found to be significantly associated with later reading achievement. The coefficients obtained for the subgroups were then compared to those for the total group. Only if the coefficients obtained for the subgroups were both substantially less than that for the total group, was the significant association assumed to be at least in part a function of intelligence.

Table I-5. D_{yx} Coefficients of Correlation Between Grade II ORP Index and Potentially Predictive Kindergarten Tests, by Sex (for children in the general sample)

Test	Boys (N = 31)	Girls (N = 22)
Correlation higher for girls		
Hyperactivity, Distractibility, and Disinhibition Index	.35	.85
Human-Figure Drawing	.16	.31
Bender Visuo-Motor Gestalt	.35	.66
Tapped Patterns	.12	.59
Auditory Discrimination (Wepman)	.12	.40
Number of Words	.18	.49
Categories	.18	.35
Letter Naming	.32	.41
Reversals (Horst)	.12	.64
Word Matching (Gates)	.22	.56
Word Rhyming (Gates)	.14	.31
Word Recognition I (Pack)	.35	.45
Ego Strength	.16	.80
Work Attitude	.39	.47
Correlation higher for boys		
Story Organization	.40	.20
Word Recognition II (Table)	.54	.38
Little difference between boys and girls		
Pencil Use	.36	.38
Name Writing	.41	.47
Word Reproduction	.46	.42

Table I-6. Performance on Grade II Achievement Tests, by Sex (per cent of children in the general sample attaining critical score level)

Test	Boys (N = 31)	Girls (N = 22)	P
Reading	26	36	$> .05$
Writing	32	41	$> .05$
Spelling	48	73	$> .05$

Table I-7. Performance on Grade II Achievement Tests, by Race
(per cent of children in the general sample attaining
critical score level)

Test	Negro (N = 21)	Caucasian (N = 32)	P
Reading	19	38	$>.05$
Writing	29	40	$>.05$
Spelling	29	59	$<.05$

Table I-8. The Effectiveness of the Predictive Index,
Grade II Achievement in Reading and Spelling, by
Predictive Index Score
(for children in the general sample)

ORP Index and Metropolitan Spelling Score	Predictive Index Score 7–10	4–6	0–3	Total
Reading advanced or better than adequate; spelling grade 3.5 or above	16	15	2	33
Reading adequate; spelling grade 2.5–3.4	1	4	2	7
Reading less than adequate or poor; spelling grade 2.4 or below		1	10	11
Total	17	20	14	51[a]

[a] Two children who did not take all ten tests are excluded from the table.

Table I-9. $D_{y.x}$ Coefficients of Correlation Between 37 Kindergarten Tests and
Grade II Achievement Tests
(for prematurely and maturely born children)

KINDERGARTEN TEST	GRADE II TEST					
	ORP Index		Writing		Spelling	
	Mature	Pre-mature	Mature	Pre-mature	Mature	Pre-mature
Behavioral patterning: Hyperactivity, Distractibility, and Disinhibition Index	.46*	.23*	.48†	.30*	.40*	.04
Motility patterning: Concomitant Movements	.03	.06	.05	.12	.04	—.06

KINDERGARTEN TEST	GRADE II TEST					
	ORP Index		Writing		Spelling	
	Mature	Pre-mature	Mature	Pre-mature	Mature	Pre-mature
Gross motor patterning:						
Balance	.09	—.06	—.15	.12	.14	—.18
Hopping	.22	.28	.18	.54†	.18	.31
Throwing	.10	.18	.06	.11	.14	.00
Fine motor patterning:						
Pegboard Speed Index	.17	.24*	.27*	.28†	.23*	.21*
Tying a Knot	.13	.26	.38	.26	—.16	.32
Pencil Use	.34*	.31*	.46†	.38†	.27	.19
Body image:						
Human-figure Drawing	.23*	.21*	.11	.35†	.20*	.20*
Laterality:						
Hand Preference Index	.10	—.01	.18	.04	.15	—.02
Visual-perceptual patterning:						
Figure-ground Organization	.05	—.02	.16	—.03	.12	.03
Bender Visuo-Motor Gestalt	.44†	.47†	.33†	.51†	.45†	.38†
Auditory-perceptual patterning:						
Tapped Patterns	.30*	.36†	.23	.34†	.36*	.36†
Auditory Memory Span	.28	.22	.29	—.02	.20	.24
Auditory Discrimination						
(Wepman)	.26*	.42†	.11	.47†	.31*	.49†
Word Recognition (Peabody)	.21	.35*	.16	.27*	.26*	.48†
Language Comprehension	.21	.33†	.06	.10	.20	.24*
Expressive Language:						
Consonant Articulation	.12	.15	.01	.28*	.03	.24*
Articulatory Stability	.16	.13	—.17	.19	.24	.11
Word Finding	.20	.33†	.18	.34†	.26	.42†
Story Organization	.28*	.19	.05	.18	.27*	.14
Number of Words	.40†	.08	.27*	.12	.32*	.08
Sentence Elaboration	.18	.04	.16	.03	.23	.09
Number of Grammatical Errors	.09	.13	.01	.03	.07	.11
Definitions (Binet)	.07	.20	.14	.38†	.10	.29*
Categories	.24*	.31*	.23*	.44†	.36*	.42†
Reading Readiness:						
Name Writing	.43†	.46†	.30*	.41†	.32*	.51†
Copying of Letters	.16	.30†	.35*	.41†	.30*	.47†
Letter Naming	.55†	.25*	.34*	.24	.56†	.31*

KINDERGARTEN TEST	GRADE II TEST					
	ORP Index		Writing		Spelling	
	Mature	Pre-mature	Mature	Pre-mature	Mature	Pre-mature
Reversals (Horst)	.36†	.35†	.25†	.27†	.34*	.34†
Word Matching (Gates)	.35†	.39†	.19*	.41†	.37*	.39†
Word Rhyming (Gates)	.22*	.42†	.13	.13	.15	.39†
Word Recognition I (Pack)	.40†	.42†	.38†	.34†	39†	.41†
Word Recognition II (Table)	.48†	.40†	.24*	.30*	.45†	.41†
Word Reproduction	.42†	.34†	.31†	.38†	.39†	.34†
Style:						
Ego Strength	.48*	.61†	.35*	.59†	.39*	.53†
Work Attitude	.43*	.26*	.38*	.38*	.46†	.11

* .01 ≤ P ≤ .05.
† P ≤ .01.

Table I-10.   Background Characteristics of Prematurely and Maturely Born Children

Background Characteristic	Per Cent of Prematures (N = 53)	Per Cent of Maturely Born (N = 53)	P
Age at time of kindergarten tests			
6 years and older	38	36	
5 years, 8 months, and younger	34	28	
Sex: Boys	47	59	
Race: Negroes	32	40	
Mother's education: Posthigh,			
school training or college	30	8	≤.01
Mother's employment status:			
Mother works	24	24	
IQ			
113–116	9	25	≤.05
84–94	26	8	≤.05

Table I-11. Performance of Prematurely Born Children on Grade I and
Grade II Achievement Tests, by Sex
(per cent of children attaining critical score level)

Test	Boys (N = 25)	Girls (N = 28)	P
Grade I			
Reading	20	43	
Writing	64	86	
Grade II			
Reading	36	57	
Writing	36	79	≤.01
Spelling	36	73	≤.05

Table I-12. Performance of Prematurely Born Children on Grade I and
Grade II Achievement Tests, by Birthweight
(per cent of children attaining critical score level)

| Test | Birthweight | | |
	1,500 Grams or Less (N = 14)	1,501–1,750 Grams (N = 22)	1,751–2,500 Grams (N = 16)
Grade I			
Reading	14	27	37
Writing	43	32	62
Grade II			
Reading	28	54	37
Writing	14	45	37
Spelling	35	59	56

Table I-13.   Performance of Prematurely and Maturely Born Children on
37 Kindergarten Tests
(per cent of children attaining critical score level)

Test	Prematures (N = 53)	Maturely Born (N = 53)	P
Behavioral patterning: Hyperactivity, Distractibility and Disinhibition	62	81	
Motility Patterning:			
Concomitant Movements	35	62	≤.01
Gross motor patterning			
Balance	87	91	
Hopping	76	89	
Throwing	80	85	
Fine motor patterning			
Pegboard Speed Index	58	81	≤.05
Tying a Knot	87	94	
Pencil Use	61	72	
Body image: Human-figure Drawing	76	89	
Laterality: Hand Preference Index	59	72	
Visual-perceptual Patterning:			
Figure-ground Organization	39	55	
Bender Visuo-Motor Gestalt	62	91	≤.01
Auditory-perceptual patterning:			
Tapped Patterns	61	93	≤.01
Auditory Memory Span	82	89	
Auditory Discrimination (Wepman)	67	81	
Word Recognition (Peabody)	74	90	≤.05
Language Comprehension	72	94	≤.01
Expressive language:			
Consonant Articulation	15	29	
Articulatory Stability	70	83	
Word Finding	83	98	≤.05
Story Organization	45	71	≤.05
Number of Words	30	47	
Sentence Elaboration	49	55	
Number of Grammatical Errors	27	10	
Definitions (Binet)	35	45	
Categories	35	59	≤.05
Reading readiness			
Name Writing	70	92	≤.01

Test	Prematures (N = 53)	Maturely Born (N = 53)	P
Copying of Letters	70	94	≤.01
Letter Naming	47[a]	78[a]	≤.05
Reversals (Horst)	33	45	
Word Matching (Gates)	50	79	≤.01
Word Rhyming (Gates)	69	85	≤.05
Word Recognition I (Pack)	37	60	≤.05
Word Recognition II (Table)	38	57	
Word Reproduction	53	72	
Style			
Ego Strength	65	81	
Work Attitude	61	74	

[a] Based on 32 prematurely and 27 maturely born children.

Table I-14.   Performance of Prematurely and Maturely Born Children on Grade I and Grade II Achievement Tests
(per cent of children attaining critical score level)

Test	Prematures (N = 53)	Maturely Born (N = 53)	P
Grade I			
Reading	34	57	≤.05
Writing	13	34	≤.01
Grade II			
Reading	47	79	≤.01
Writing	58	79	≤.05
Spelling	55	77	≤.05

Table I-15. Rate of Progress from Kindergarten to Grade II of Prematurely
and Maturely Born Children
(per cent of children attaining critical score level on four nonacademic tests)

Test	Prematures (N = 53)	Maturely Born (N = 53)
Laterality Index		
Kindergarten	59	71
Grade II	66	65
Net degree of progress or regression[a]	+.17	—.08
Bender Visuo-Motor Gestalt Test		
Kindergarten	46[b]	66[b]
Grade II	39[b]	59[b]
Net degree of progress or regression[a]	—.15	—.11
Auditory Discrimination		
Kindergarten	30[b]	55[b]
Grade II	81[b]	86[b]
Net degree of progress or regression[a]	+.73	+.69
Behavioral Index		
Kindergarten	64	81
Grade II	71	77
Net degree of progress or regression[d]	+.19	—.05

[a] The net degree of progress (+) or regression (—) is the ratio of the actual change to the maximum possible change, taking into account that the prematures, starting from a lower level, could achieve greater absolute improvement. The Laterality Index illustrates the calculations:

Net progress of prematures = actual progress ÷ maximum progress possible = (66% — 59%) ÷ (100% — 59%) = +.17.

Net regression of maturely born = actual regression ÷ maximum regression possible = (65% — 71%) ÷ (71% — 0%) = —.08.

[b] Based on 33 prematurely and 29 maturely born children who were born in 1956. The Bender-Gestalt and Auditory Discrimination tests were not readministered to children born in 1955.

Table I-16. Absolute Performance of Prematurely and Maturely Born Children
on Four Kindergarten Tests Readministered at Grade II
(per cent of children attaining critical score level)

Test	Prematures (N = 53)	Maturely Born (N = 53)	P
Laterality Index	74	83	
Bender-Gestalt	67[a]	93[a]	≦.05
Auditory Discrimination	73[a]	79[a]	
Behavioral Index	71	77	

[a] Based on 33 prematurely and 29 maturely born children who were born in 1956.
The Bender-Gestalt and Auditory Discrimination tests were not readministered to
children born in 1955.

Table I-17. Performance of Children in the General Sample on
37 Kindergarten Tests, by Age at Kindergarten Testing
(per cent of children attaining critical score level)
Identification of "Maturation-Sensitive" Tests

Tests, Listed According to Sensitivity to Maturation	5 Yrs., 8 Mos., and Below (N = 15)	5 Yrs., 9 Mos., to 5 Yrs., 11 Mos. (N = 19)	6 Yrs., 0 Mos., and Above (N = 19)
Consistently maturation-sensitive			
Balance	87	90	95
Pegboard Speed Index	20	32	47
Pencil Use	67	68	79
Hand Preference Index	53	74	84
Tapped Patterns	27	32	42
Auditory Discrimination			
(Wepman)	7	16	26
Word Recognition (Peabody)	7	26	37
Story Organization	27	32	53
Definitions (Binet)	27	47	58
Name Writing	53	53	84
Letter Naming	0	40	73
Word Recognition I (Pack)	47	58	74
Word Recognition II (Table)	40	63	63
Word Reproduction	27	47	68
Ego Strength	73	78	90

Tests, Listed According to Sensitivity to Maturation	5 Yrs., 8 Mos., and Below (N = 15)	5 Yrs., 9 Mos., to 5 Yrs., 11 Mos. (N = 19)	6 Yrs., 0 Mos., and Above (N = 19)
Maturation-sensitive to a lesser degree			
Concomitant Movements	60	53	74
Bender Visuo-Motor Gestalt	53	47	79
Number of Words	40	37	65
Sentence Elaboration	40	37	88
Categories	53	53	68
Copying of Letters	60	53	79
Reversals (Horst)	27	5	47
Word Matching (Gates)	46	42	74
Word Rhyming (Gates)	47	43	69
Work Attitude	73	68	79
Not maturation-sensitive			
Hyperactivity, Distractibility, and Disinhibition	80	84	79
Hopping	93	84	90
Throwing	93	74	90
Tying a Knot	100	84	100
Human-figure Drawing	33	16	37
Figure-ground Organization	60	47	58
Auditory Memory Span	93	84	90
Language Comprehension	73	68	68
Consonant Articulation	40	22	28
Articulatory Stability	73	100	74
Word Finding	73	63	63
Number of Grammatical Errors	40	31	18

Table I-18. Number of Predictive and Not Predictive Kindergarten Tests in Maturation and Not Maturation-Sensitive Categories

Tests	Relation to Maturation		
	Maturation-Sensitive	Not Maturation-Sensitive	Total
Predictive	19	2	21
Not Predictive	6	10	16
Total	25	12	37

Appendix II

Administering and Scoring the
Predictive Index Tests

◆

PENCIL USE

The child is observed as he uses the pencil.

The score, from best to worst, ranges from 0–2. The child is penalized one point if his grasp is so loose that he can hardly hold the pencil. He is penalized two points if he is entirely unable to manipulate the pencil or if he presses so hard that he tears the page.

BENDER VISUO-MOTOR GESTALT TEST

The child is asked to copy six (A, 1, 2, 4, 6, and 8) of the nine designs.

Ability to perceive and respond to the essentials of the Gestalten and degree of differentiation are evaluated. Criteria were discussed with Dr. Lauretta Bender (14).

Instructions

"Here are some designs for you to copy. Just copy them the way you see them."

Score

The score is the number of copies, from 0–6, on which the child fails to reproduce the essential features of the Gestalt. One point is added if he is unable to arrange the designs on paper—if, for instance, designs are superimposed on one another. Another point is added if he rotates three or more of the figures.

WEPMAN AUDITORY DISCRIMINATION TEST

The twenty odd-numbered word-pairs from this test are presented, and the child is asked to indicate whether the words in each pair sound the "same" or "different." Some children require extensive practice in order to grasp and apply this concept.

Instructions

"I am going to say two words. I want you to tell me whether I say the same word twice or whether I say two different words. Try this: hand-sand. Did I say the same word twice? You're right, I said two *different* words: 'hand' is not the same as 'sand.' Now try this: month-month. You're right, I said the same word two times. Now listen to the words I'm going to say and tell me if they sound the same or different. Turn your chair around so you cannot see me. I want to see how well you can listen."

Score

The child's score, from 0–15, is the number of errors on dissimilar pairs (X-errors).

NUMBER OF WORDS USED IN A STORY

The number of words the child uses in telling the story of *The Three Bears* is counted. The definition of what constitutes a word is taken from Edith Davis (50): Contractions of subject and predicate, like "it's" and "we're" are counted as two words; contractions of the verb and the negative, such as "can't" are considered to be one word; each part of a verbal combination is taken as a separate word: thus "have been playing" are three words; hyphenated and compound nouns—"oh boy," "all right," and so forth—are counted as *one* word.

Score

The total number of words used by the child constitutes the score.

CATEGORIES

Each child is asked to produce class names for three groups of words: colors (red-green-blue), boys (Tom-Charley-Henry), and food (apple-hamburger-ice cream).

Instructions

"What are these things: red-green-blue?" (If the child does not respond correctly, continue: "I'll tell you about three other things: ball-doll-marbles. They're *all* toys. Now tell me what are red-green-blue?) What are Tom-Charley-Henry? And what are apple-hamburger-ice cream?"

Score

The score, from 0–3, is the number of categories missed.

HORST REVERSALS TEST

The particular section of the Horst Reversals Test used consists of ten rows* of two- and three-letter combinations, presented in correct and reversed order, which have to be matched to a model. The first row is used for purposes of demonstration and the nine remaining rows are administered.

ot	to. ot . ot . to ot . to
de	de . ed . de . ed . ed . de
ɹɑ	ɑɹ . ɑɹ . ɹɑ . ɹɑ . ɑɹ . ɑɹ
nu	nu . un . un . nu . un
pot	top . pot . pot . top
bad	bad . dab . dab . bad
les	sel . les . les . sel
pik	pik . kip . kip . pik
sof	fos . sof . sof . fos
man	nam . nam . man . man

* The original section of the test consists of twelve rows of which lines four and five were omitted to save time.

Instructions

Since this test is difficult, it may prove necessary to provide considerable help. The examiner shields all but the first row and points to the model. "Tell me which one looks exactly like the one I have my finger on. Now you find another." If the child does not understand, the examiner says, pointing to the model, "You see, some of them are backwards, the others are the right way. Pick out those that look like the one I have my finger on." The shield is removed after the second row has been attempted. The examiners need not hesitate to point to configurations to help the child keep his place. Assistance is provided as long as the child seems to benefit, but is discontinued if the task is clearly too difficult.

Score

A child's score, from 0–9, consists of the number of *rows* in which he makes errors in matching.

GATES WORD-MATCHING SUBTESTS

Each child is asked to do twelve of the eighteen exercises from the Word-Matching subtest of the Gates Reading Readiness battery. The twelve exercises used are (reading in rows from left to right): 2, 3, 4, 5, 8, 9, 10, 11, 14, 15, 16, and 17. The first exercise is used for demonstration.

Instructions

The examiner shields all but the first exercise, saying, "There are two words in this box which look exactly alike. Can you find them? Take your pencil and draw a line between the ones that look the same. Now *you* do the next one by yourself." If the child fails to understand what is required, the examiner clarifies the task. The shield is removed after the child completes exercises 2 and 3.

Score

The number of mistakes, from 0–12, is the child's score.

WORD RECOGNITION I AND II
AND WORD REPRODUCTION

The words "boy" and "train," written on separate index cards, are shown to each child at the beginning of the testing session. He is taught to recognize and say these words when they are presented one after the other and when they are placed side by side on the table. When the examiner is convinced that the child is, at least for the moment, able to "read" them, he asks the subject to *copy* the words on lined paper. About half way through the session both words are re-exposed and studied. At the end of the session the following three tests are administered:

Word Recognition I

The words "boy" and "train" are placed in third and seventh position among a pack of ten words. These ten words are presented one after another, and the child is asked to point to "boy" and "train" when he encounters them.

Instructions

"Remember the two words you learned to read? What were they?" (If the child fails to remember the words, they are supplied.) "I've put 'boy' and 'train' in this pack with some other words. Point to 'boy' and 'train' when you see them."

Word Reproduction II

The same words are exposed in rows on the table, and the child is asked to pick out "boy" and "train."

Score

The child's score on each of the two tests is the number of times, from 0–2, he fails to identify the two words previously taught.

Word Reproduction

The child is required to write as much as he can remember of the words "boy" and "train."

Instructions

The words "boy" and "train" are again exposed, and the child is asked to remember the way they look. The words are then removed, and the examiner says, "Now write the words 'boy' and 'train' the way you did when you first came."

Score

Each word is scored from 0–3, according to the number of letters written down correctly.

boy
3   word spelled perfectly
2   two letters of the word reproduced
1   one letter reproduced
0   failure to recall any letter

train
3   word spelled perfectly
2   three or four letters of the word reproduced
1   one or two letters reproduced
0   failure to recall any letter

The final score, from 0–6, is the sum of scores for each word. Letter reversals are not counted as errors. However, if letter order is confused, or if letters are added, one point is subtracted from the child's score.

ADMINISTERING AND SCORING
OF END-OF-SECOND-GRADE TESTS

Gates Advanced Primary Reading Test, Gray Oral Reading Test, Metropolitan Spelling Test

These tests are administered and scored according to procedures outlined in the manuals.

The Writing Test

Each child is asked to write four sentences to dictation. The sentences consist in large part of words taken from the Metropolitan Spelling Test.

Score

The score ranges from 0–4.

If the child's writing is adequate for end of second grade, that is to say, if rhythm and flow reflect his understanding of the sentence, he receives a score of 0. One point is added if individual letters are distorted or reversed; another point if words are omitted, or if the child is unable to hold to the line, or if words run into each other. One or two further points are added according to the degree to which the child fails to integrate single letters into a cohesive word.

Appendix III

Critical Score Levels

◆

The critical score levels presented in Table III-1 represent the score levels that gave maximum differentiation between the children who failed in reading and the rest of the subjects. The value shown is the lowest a child could have scored and still have attained the critical score level.

Table III-1. Critical Score Levels on 10 Kindergarten Tests Included in the Predictive Index[a]

Test	Score Range (best—poorest)	Critical Score Level
Pencil Use	0–2	0 (Level expected for age)
Bender Visuo-Motor Gestalt (A, 1, 2, 4, 6, 8)	0–6	1 (At least 5 designs copied correctly)
Auditory Discrimination (Wepman)	0–11	1 X-error
Number of Words	594–54	226 words
Categories	0–3	0 (All series correctly categorized)
Reversals (Horst)	0–9	4 (At least 5 rows correctly matched)
Word Matching (Gates)	0–12	3 (At least 9 words correctly paired)
Word Recognition I (Pack)	0–2	0 (Both words identified)
Word Recognition II (Table)	0–2	0 (Both words identified)
Word Reproduction	6–0	3 (See scoring system in Appendix II)

[a] See Table I-8.

References Cited

●

1. Ajuriaguerra, Julian de. "Les Désordres du Langage chez l'Enfant." Paper read at the Conference on Speech, Language and Communication at the Brain Research Institute, University of California, Los Angeles, November 1963.
2. Ajuriaguerra, Julian de, and Hecaen, Henry. *Les Gauchers, Prévalence Manuelle et Dominance Cérébrale.* Paris: Presses Universitaires de France, 1963.
3. Anderson, Virgil A. *Improving the Child's Speech.* New York: Oxford University Press, 1953.
4. Arnold, Godfrey. "Signs and Symptoms," in *Studies in Tachyphemia.* New York: Speech Rehabilitation Institute, 1964.
5. Artley, A. Sterl. "A Study of Certain Factors Presumed to Be Associated with Reading and Speech Difficulties," *Journal of Speech and Hearing Disorders,* 13 (1948), 351–360.
6. Austin, Mary C., and Morrison, Coleman. *The First R: The Harvard Report on Reading in Elementary Schools.* New York: Macmillan, 1963.
7. Barber, Lucille. "Immature Ego Development as a Factor in Retarded Ability to Read." Ph.D. thesis, University of Michigan, 1952.
8. Barrett, Thomas C. "Visual Discrimination Tasks as Predictors of First Grade Reading Achievement," *Reading Teacher,* 18 (1965), 276–282.
9. Beckett, Dorothy. "Philosophical Differences in Reading Concepts," *Reading Teacher,* 18 (1964), 27–32.
10. Bender, Lauretta. "The Goodenough Test (Drawing-a-Man) in Chronic Encephalitis in Children," *Quarterly Journal of Child Behavior,* 3 (1951), 449–459.

11. ———. *Psychopathology of Children with Organic Brain Disorders.* Springfield, Ill.: Chas. C. Thomas, 1956.

12. ———. "Problems in Conceptualization and Communication in Children with Developmental Alexia," in P. Hoch and J. Zubin (eds.), *Psychopathology of Communication.* New York: Grune & Stratton, 1958.

13. ———. "Mental Illness in Childhood and Heredity," *Eugenics Quarterly*, 10 (1963), 1–11.

14. ———. "The Visual Motor Gestalt Function in Six and Seven Year Old Normal, Schizophrenic, and Brain Damaged Children." Paper presented at the Meeting of the American Psychopathological Association, New York, February 1966.

15. ———. "Plasticity in Developmental Neurology and Psychiatry," in P. Hoch and J. Zubin (eds.), *Schizophrenia.* New York: Grune & Stratton, 1966.

16. Benton, Arthur L. "Mental Development of Prematurely Born Children: A Critical Review of the Literature," *American Journal of Orthopsychiatry*, 10 (1940), 719–746.

17. ———. "Dyslexia in Relation to Form Perception and Directional Sense," in J. Money (ed.), *Reading Disability, Progress and Research Needs in Dyslexia.* Baltimore: Johns Hopkins Press, 1962.

18. Bentzen, Frances. "Sex Ratios in Learning and Behavior," *American Journal of Orthopsychiatry*, 33 (1963), 92–98.

19. Betts, Emmett A. *The Prevention and Correction of Reading Difficulties.* Evanston, Ill.: Row, Peterson & Co., 1936.

20. Birch, Herbert G., and Belmont, Lillian. "Lateral Dominance, Lateral Awareness, and Reading Disability," *Child Development*, 36 (1965), 57–71.

21. ———. "Auditory-Visual Integration, Intelligence and Reading Ability in School Children," *Perceptual and Motor Skills*, 20 (1965), 295–305.

22. Blanchard, Phyllis. "Psychoanalytic Contributions to Problems of Reading Disability," *Psychoanalytic Study of the Child*, 2 (1946), 163–187.

23. Blau, Abram, *et al.* "The Psychogenic Etiology of Premature Birth," *Psychosomatic Medicine*, 25 (1963), 201–211.

24. Blegen, Sigrid. "The Premature Child," *Acta Paediatrica*, Supplement 88 (1952).

25. Borel-Maisonny, Suzanne. "Les Troubles du Langage dans les Dyslexies et les Dysorthographies," *Enfance*, 4 (1951), 400–444.

26. ———. "La Dyslexie et sa Prévention," *Réadaptation*, 58 (1959), 15–20.

27. Bradley, Charles. "Organic Factors in the Psychopathology of Childhood," in P. Hoch and J. Zubin (eds.), *Psychopathology of Childhood*. New York: Grune & Stratton, 1955.

28. Bryant, N. Dale. "Reading Disability: Part of a Syndrome of Neurological Dysfunctioning," in J. Allen Figurel (ed.), *Challenge and Experiment in Reading. Conference Proceedings of the International Reading Association*, 7 (1962), 139–143.

29. ———. "Some Conclusions Concerning Impaired Motor Development among Reading Disability Cases," *Bulletin of the Orton Society*, 14 (1964), 16–17.

30. ———. "Some Principles of Remedial Instruction for Dyslexia," *Reading Teacher*, 18 (1965), 567–572.

31. Burks, Harold F. "The Effect on Learning of Brain Pathology," *Exceptional Children*, 24 (1957), 169–172.

32. ———. "The Hyperkinetic Child," *Exceptional Children*, 27 (1960), 18–26.

33. Byrne, Margaret. "The Wepman Auditory Discrimination Test as a Clinical Tool." Paper presented at the Annual Meeting of the American Speech and Hearing Association, New York, 1962.

34. Carroll, John B. *The Study of Language*. Cambridge: Harvard University Press, 1953.

35. ———. "Language Development," in *Encyclopedia of Educational Research*. New York: Macmillan, 1960, pp. 744–752.

36. Carson, Arnold S., and Rabin, A. J. "Verbal Comprehension and Communication in Negro and White Children," *Journal of Educational Psychology*, 51 (1960), 47–51.

37. Castner, B. M. "Prediction of Reading Disability Prior to First Grade Entrance," *American Journal of Orthopsychiatry*, 5 (1935), 375–387.

38. Centeno, Pilar A., Walter, Ruth, and Thelander, H. E. "A Five-Year Study of Prematurity," *California Medicine*, 84 (1956), 269–278.

39. Chall, Jeanne, *et al.* "Language, Visual, Auditory and Visual-Motor Factors in Beginning Reading: A Preliminary Analysis."

Paper presented at meeting of the American Educational Research Association, Chicago, February 1965.

40. Chess, Stella. "Developmental Language Disability as a Factor in Personality Distortion in Childhood," *American Journal of Orthopsychiatry*, 14 (1944), 483–490.

41. Cleland, Donald L. "Seeing and Reading," *American Journal of Optometry*, 30 (1953), 467–481.

42. Cohen, Theodore B. "Diagnostic and Predictive Methods with Young Children," *American Journal of Orthopsychiatry*, 33 (1963), 330–331.

43. Cohn, Robert. "Delayed Acquisition of Reading and Writing Abilities in Children," *Archives of Neurology*, 4 (1961), 153–164.

44. Cole, Edwin. "Specific Reading Disability. A Problem in Integration and Adaptation," *American Journal of Ophthalmology*, 34 (1951), 226–232.

45. Coleman, J. M., Iscoe, Ira, and Brodsky, Marvin. "The Draw-a-Man Test as a Predictor of School Readiness and as an Index of Emotional and Physical Maturity," *Pediatrics*, 24 (1959), 275–281.

46. Coleman, Richard, and Deutsch, Cynthia. "Lateral Dominance and Right-Left Discrimination: A Comparison of Normal and Retarded Readers," *Perceptual and Motor Skills*, 19 (1964), 43–50.

47. Critchley, Macdonald. *Developmental Dyslexia*. London: Wm. Heinemann Medical Books, 1964.

48. Cruickshank, William, *et al*. *A Teaching Method for Brain-Injured and Hyperactive Children*. Syracuse, N. Y.: Syracuse University Press, 1961.

49. Darley, Frederick L., and Moll, Kenneth L. "Reliability of Language Measures and Size of Language Sample," *Journal of Speech and Hearing Research*, 3 (1960), 166–173.

50. Davis, Edith. "The Development of Linguistic Skills in Twins, Singletons with Siblings, and Only Children from Age Five to Ten Years," *University of Minnesota Child Welfare Monograph*, Series XIV (1937), p. 44.

51. Davis, Irene P. "The Speech Aspects of Reading Readiness," in *National Education Association*, Department of Elementary School Principals, 17th Yearbook (1938), 282–289.

52. Deutsch, Cynthia. "Auditory Discrimination and Learning: Social Factors." Arden House Conference on Pre-School Enrichment of Socially Disadvantaged Children, December 1962.

53. Deutsch, Martin. "Minority-Group and Class Status, as Related to Social and Personality Factors in Scholastic Achievement," *Society for Applied Anthropology*, Monograph 2 (1960).

54. ———. "Facilitating Development in the Pre-School Child: Social and Psychological Perspectives." Arden House Conference on Pre-School Enrichment of Socially Disadvantaged Children, December 1962. Published in *Merrill-Palmer Quarterly of Behavior and Development*, 10 (1964), 249–263.

55. ———. "The Role of Social Class in Language Development and Cognition," *American Journal of Orthopsychiatry*, 35 (1965), 78–88.

56. Diack, Hunter. *Reading and the Psychology of Perception.* Nottingham, England: Peter Skinner Publishing Co., 1960.

57. Douglas, J. W. B. "Mental Ability and School Achievement of Premature Children at 8 Years of Age," *British Medical Journal*, I, 4977 (1956), 1210–1214.

58. ———. "Premature Children at Primary Schools," *British Medical Journal*, 5178 (1960), 1008–1013.

59. Drew, Arthur L. "A Neurological Appraisal of Familial Congenital Word Blindness," *Brain*, 79 (1956), 440–460.

60. Drillien, Cecil M. *The Growth and Development of the Prematurely Born Infant.* Baltimore: Williams & Wilkins, 1964.

61. Dunn, Lloyd M. *Peabody Picture Vocabulary Test.* Nashville, Tenn.: American Guidance Service, 1959.

62. Durrell, Donald D. "First-Grade Reading Success Study: A Summary," *Journal of Education*, 140 (1958), 1–6.

63. Eisenberg, Leon, and Gruenberg, Ernest. "The Current Status of Secondary Prevention in Child Psychiatry," *American Journal of Orthopsychiatry*, 31 (1961), 355–367.

64. Escalona, Sibylle, and Heider, Grace. *Prediction and Outcome.* New York: Basic Books, 1959.

65. Fabian, Abraham A. "Clinical and Experimental Studies of School Children Who Are Retarded in Reading," *Quarterly Journal of Child Behavior*, 3 (1951), 15–37.

66. Fernald, Grace. *Remedial Techniques in Basic School Subjects.* New York: McGraw-Hill, 1945.

67. Fite, June H., and Schwartz, Louise A. "Screening Culturally Disadvantaged First-Grade Children for Potential Reading Difficulties due to Constitutional Factors," *American Journal of Orthopsychiatry*, 35 (1965), 359–360.

68. Freedman, Alfred M., *et al.* "The Influence of Hyperbilirubinemia on the Early Development of the Premature," Psychiatric Research Report, *American Psychiatric Association*, 13 (1960), 108–127.

69. Freeman, Frank. *Guiding Growth in Handwriting, Evaluation Scale.* Columbus, Ohio: Parker Zaner-Bloser Co., 1958.

70. French, Edward L. "Psychological Factors in Cases of Reading Difficulties." Paper presented at the Twenty-seventh Annual Conference of the Secondary Educational Board, New York, 1953.

71. Freud, Anna. *Normality and Pathology in Childhood.* New York: International Universities Press, 1965.

72. Freud, Sigmund. *On Aphasia.* New York: International Universities Press, 1953.

73. Frostig, Marianne. *Developmental Test of Visual Perception.* Palo Alto, Calif.: Consulting Psychologists Press.

74. Galton, Francis. *Inquiries into the Human Faculty and Its Development.* New York: Macmillan, 1883.

75. Gates, Arthur. "The Role of Personality Maladjustment in Reading Disability," *Journal of Genetic Psychology*, 59 (1941), 77–83.

76. Gallagher, J. Roswell. "Specific Language Disability (Dyslexia)," *Clinical Proceedings, Children's Hospital, Washington, D.C.*, 16 (1960), 3–15.

77. Gavel, Sylvia. "June Reading Achievement of First Grade Children," *Journal of Education*, 140 (1958), 37–43.

78. Gesell, Arnold. *The Mental Growth of the Pre-School Child.* New York: Macmillan, 1930.

79. ———. *The First Five Years of Life.* New York: Harper & Row, 1940.

80. ———. *The Embryology of Behavior—The Beginning of the Human Mind.* New York: Harper & Row, 1945.

81. Gibson, Eleanor. "Association and Differentiation in Perceptual Learning." Unpublished paper, Cornell University, 1961.

82. Goins, Jean Turner. "Visual Perception Abilities and Early Reading Progress." *Supplementary Educational Monograph*, 87 (1958). Chicago: University of Chicago Press.

83. Goldberg, Herman, "The Ophthalmologist Looks at the Reading Problem," *American Journal of Ophthalmology*, 47 (1959), 67–74.

84. Goldstein, Raphael. "The Problem of Reading Disabilities," *Clinical Pediatrics*, 3 (1964), 105–107.

85. Greenacre, Phyllis. *Trauma, Growth and Personality*. London: Hogarth Press, 1953.

86. Grewel, Frits. "How Do Children Acquire Use of Language?" *Phonetica*, 3 (1959), 193–202.

87. ———. Personal communication.

88. Gutelius, Margaret F., and Layman, Emma M. "Reading Disability, or Developmental Dyslexia," *Clinical Proceedings, Children's Hospital, Washington, D.C.*, 16 (1960), 15–27.

89. Hall, R. Vance. "Does Entrance Age Affect Achievement?" *Elementary School Journal*, 63 (1963), 391–396.

90. Hallgren, Bertil. "Specific Dyslexia: A Clinical and Genetic Study," *Acta Psychiatrica et Neurologica*, Supplement 65 (1950).

91. Hardy, William. "Dyslexia in Relation to Diagnostic Methodology in Hearing and Speech Disorders," in J. Money (ed.), *Reading Disability, Progress and Research Needs in Dyslexia*. Baltimore: Johns Hopkins Press, 1962.

92. Harper, Paul A. Personal communication, April 1964.

93. Harper, Paul A., Fischer, Liselotte K., and Rider, Rowland V. "Neurological and Intellectual Status of Prematures at Three to Five Years of Age," *Journal of Pediatrics*, 55 (1959), 679–690.

94. Harrington, Sister Mary James, and Durrell, Donald D. "Mental Maturity vs. Perception Abilities in Primary Reading," *Journal of Educational Psychology*, 46 (1955), 375–380.

95. Harris, Albert J. "Lateral Dominance, Directional Confusion and Reading Disability," *Journal of Psychology*, 44 (1957), 283–294.

96. ———. "Visual and Auditory Perception in Learning to Read," *Optometric Weekly*, 50 (1959), 2115–2121.

97. ———. *How to Increase Reading Ability*. New York: Longmans, Green, 1961.

98. Harris, Irving D. *Emotional Blocks to Learning*. Glencoe, Ill.: The Free Press, 1961.

99. Hartmann, Heinz, Kris, Ernst, and Loewenstein, Rudolph M. "Papers on Psychoanalytic Psychology," *Psychological Issues*, 4 (1964), No. 2.

100. Hawke, William. "Specific Reading Disabilities," *Pediatric Clinics of North America*, (1958), 513–522.

101. Hebb, Donald O. *Organization of Behavior*. New York: Wiley, 1949.

102. Hejna, Robert Frank. *Developmental Articulation Test*. Madison, Wis.: College Printing & Typing Co., 1955.

103. Hendrick, Ives. *Facts and Theories of Psychoanalysis*. London: Kegan Paul, 1934.

104. Henig, Max S. "Predictive Value of a Reading Readiness Test and of Teachers' Forecasts," *Elementary School Journal*, 50 (1949), 41–46.

105. Hermann, Knud. *Reading Disability: A Medical Study of Word-Blindness and Related Handicaps*, Springfield, Ill.: Chas. C. Thomas, 1959.

106. Hermann, Knud, and Norrie, Edith. "Is Congenital Word-Blindness a Hereditary Type of Gerstmann's Syndrome," *Psychiatria et Neurologia* (Basel), 136 (1958), 59–73.

107. Hermann, Knud, and Voldby, H. "The Morphology of Handwriting in Congenital Word-Blindness," *Acta Psychiatrica et Neurologica*, 21 (1946), 349–363.

108. Hildreth, Gertrude. "Linguistic Factors in Early Reading Instruction," *Reading Teacher*, 18 (1964), 172–178.

109. de Hirsch, Katrina. "Specific Dyslexia or Strephosymbolia," *Folia Phoniatrica*, 4 (1952), 231–248.

110. ———. "Gestalt Psychology as Applied to Language Disturbances," *Journal of Nervous and Mental Disorders*, 120 (1954), 257–261.

111. ———. "Tests Designed to Discover Potential Reading Difficulties at the Six-Year-Old Level," *American Journal of Orthopsychiatry*, 27 (1957), 566–576.

112. ———. "Studies in Tachyphemia: IV. Diagnosis of Developmental Language Disorders," *Logos*, 4 (1961), 3–9.

113. ———. "Concepts Related to Normal Reading Processes and Their Application to Reading Pathology," *Journal of Genetic Psychology*, 102 (1963), 277–285.

114. ———. "Two Categories of Learning Difficulties in Adolescents," *American Journal of Orthopsychiatry*, 33 (1963), 87–91.

115. ———. "The Concept of Plasticity and Language Disabilities," *Speech Pathology and Therapy*, 8 (1965), 12–17.

116. Holmes, Jack A. "The Substrata-Factor Theory of Reading: Some Experimental Evidence," in J. Allen Figurel (ed.), *New Frontiers in Reading, Conference Proceedings of the International Reading Association*, 5 (1960), 115–121.

117. House, Ralph W. "A Physiological Approach to the Diagnosis of Pupils with Reading Difficulties," *Peabody Journal of Education*, 20 (1943), 294–299.

118. Ilg, Frances, and Ames, Louise. *School Readiness*. New York: Harper & Row, 1964.

119. Ingram, Thomas T. S. "Delayed Development of Speech with Special Reference to Dyslexia," *Proceedings of the Royal Society of Medicine*, 56 (1963), 199–203.

120. Izmuzi, Hisa. "Studies of Premature Children," *Japanese Journal of Educational Psychology*, 11 (1963), 43–47.

121. Jansky, Jeannette. "Congenitally Word Deaf Children." M.S. thesis, Department of Education, College of the City of New York, January 1960.

122. ———. "A Case of Severe Dyslexia with Aphasic-Like Symptoms," *Reading Teacher*, 15 (1961), 110–113.

123. Johnson, Marjorie. "A Study of Diagnostic and Remedial Procedures in a Reading Clinic Laboratory School," *Journal of Educational Research*, 48 (1955), 565–578.

124. Johnson, Marjorie, and Kress, Roy. "Philadelphia's Educational Improvement Program," *Reading Teacher*, 18 (1965), 488.

125. Kagan, Jerome. "The Child's Sex Role Classification of School Objects," *Child Development*, 35 (1964), 151–156.

126. Kainz, Friedrich. *Psychologie der Sprache. Vierter Band, Spezielle Sprachpsychologie*. Stuttgart: Ferdinand Enke Verlag, 1956.

127. Kaplan, David, and Mason, Edward. "Maternal Reactions to Premature Birth Viewed as an Acute Emotional Disorder," *Americal Journal of Orthopsychiatry*, 30 (1960), 539–547.

128. Karlin, Robert. "Physical Growth and Success in Undertaking Beginning Reading," *Journal of Educational Research*, 51 (1957), 191–201.

129. Kastein, Shulamith, and Fowler, Edmund P. "Language Development Among Survivors of Premature Birth," *A.M.A. Archives of Otolaryngology*, 69 (1959), 131–135.

130. Katan, Anny. "Some Thoughts About the Role of Verbalization

in Early Childhood," *The Psychoanalytic Study of the Child,* 16 (1961), 184–188.

131. Kawi, Ali, and Pasamanick, Benjamin. "Association of Factors of Pregnancy with Reading Disorders in Childhood," *Journal of American Medical Association,* 166 (1958), 1420–1423.

132. Keller, E. Duwayne, and Rowley, Vinton N. "Anxiety, Intelligence and Scholastic Achievement in Elementary School Children," *Psychological Reports,* 11 (1962), 19–22.

133. Keller, Suzanne. "The Social World of the Urban Slum Child," *American Journal of Orthopsychiatry,* 32 (1962) 255–256.

134. Kendall, Maurice G. *Rank Correlation Methods.* New York: Hafner, 1955.

135. Kephart, Newell. *The Slow Learner in the Classroom.* Columbus, Ohio: Charles E. Merrill Books, 1960.

136. Kermoian, Samuel B. "Teacher Appraisal of First Grade Readiness," *Elementary English,* 39 (1962), 196–201.

137. Kirk, Samuel A., and McCarthy, James J. "The Illinois Test of Psycho-Linguistic Abilities—An Approach to Differential Diagnosis," *American Journal of Mental Deficiency,* 66 (1961), 399–412.

138. Knehr, Charles, and Sobol, Albert. "Mental Ability of Prematurely Born Children at Early School Age," *Journal of Psychology,* 27 (1949), 355–361.

139. Knobloch, Hilda, and Pasamanick, Benjamin. "Environmental Factors Affecting Human Development Before and After Birth," *Pediatrics,* 26 (1960), 210–218.

140. ———. "Mental Subnormality," *New England Journal of Medicine,* 266 (1962), 1045–1051, 1092–1097, 1155–1161.

141. Koch, Helen L. "A Study of Twins Born at Different Levels of Maturity," *Child Development,* 35 (1964), 1265–1282.

142. Koffka, Kurt. *The Growth of the Mind.* London: Kegan Paul, 1928.

143. Koppitz, Elizabeth M. *The Bender Gestalt Test for Young Children.* New York: Grune & Stratton, 1964.

144. Langford, William. Personal communication.

145. Langman, Muriel Potter. "The Reading Process: A Descriptive Interdisciplinary Approach," *Genetic Psychology Monographs,* 62 (1960).

146. Lashley, Karl S. "The Problem of Serial Order in Behavior," in

L. A. Jeffress (ed.), *Cerebral Mechanisms in Behavior.* New York: Wiley, 1954.

147. Laufer, Maurice W., and Denhoff, Eric. "Hyperkinetic Behavior Syndrome," *Journal of Pediatrics,* 50 (1957), 465–474.

148. Launderville, Sister Mary Flavian. "A Study of the Effectiveness of a First-Grade Listening Test as a Predictor of Reading Achievement." Ph.D. thesis, State University of Iowa, 1958. *Abstracts,* 19 (1959), 3172–3173.

149. Lawrence, Margaret. "Minimal Brain Injury in Child Psychiatry," *Comprehensive Psychiatry,* 1 (1960), 360–369.

150. Leton, Donald A. "Visual-Motor Capacities and Ocular Efficiency in Reading," *Perceptual and Motor Skills,* 15 (1962), 407–432.

151. Levine, S. Z., and Dann, Margaret. "Survival Rates and Weight Gains in Premature Infants Weighing 1000 Grams or Less," *Annales Paediatriae Fenniae,* 3 (1957), 185–192.

152. Liss, Edward. "The Dynamics of Learning," *Quarterly Journal of Child Behavior,* 2 (1950), 140–148.

153. Lubchenco, Lula O., *et al.* "Sequelae of Premature Birth," *American Journal of Diseases of Children,* 106 (1963), 101–115.

154. McCarthy, Dorothea. "The Language Development of the Preschool Child," *University of Minnesota Child Welfare Monograph,* No. 4 (1930).

155. ―――. "Language Development in Children," in L. Carmichael (ed.), *Manual of Child Psychology.* New York: Wiley, 1954.

156. ―――. "Affective Aspects of Language Learning." Presidential address, Division of Developmental Psychology, American Psychological Association, 1961.

157. McGovney, Margarita. "Spelling Deficiency in Children of Superior General Ability," *Elementary English Review,* 7 (1930), 146–148.

158. McGraw, Mildred B. *The Neuromuscular Maturation of the Human Infant.* New York: Columbia University Press, 1943.

159. Malmquist, Eve. "Organizing Instruction to Prevent Reading Disability," in J. Allen Figurel (ed.), *Reading as an Intellectual Activity. Conference Proceedings of the International Reading Association,* 8 (1963), 36–39.

160. Martin, Clyde. "Developmental Interrelationships Among Language Variables in Children of First Grade," *Elementary English,* 32 (1955), 167–171.

161. Masland, Mary W., and Case, Linda. "Limitation of Auditory Memory as a Factor in Delayed Language Development." Paper read at Meeting of the International Association for Logopedics and Phoniatrics, Vienna, August 1965. In print.

162. Masland, Richard. "The Neurologic Substrata of Communicative Disorders." Paper read at Convention Program of the American Speech and Hearing Association, Chicago, November 1965. Not yet published in its final form.

163. Masson, J. "Exposé du Problème," *Liaison*, Numéro Spécial (1963), 21–26.

164. Menyuk, Paula. "Syntactic Structures in the Language of Children," *Journal of Child Development*, 34 (1963), 407–422.

165. Moe, Iver L. "Auding as a Predictive Measure of Reading Performance in Primary Grades." Ed.D. thesis, University of Florida, 1957. *Abstract*, 18 (1958), 121–122.

166. Monroe, Marion. "Reading Aptitude Tests for the Prediction of Success and Failure in Beginning Reading," *Education*, 56 (1935), 7–14.

167. Morgan, Elmer F., Jr. "Efficacy of Two Tests in Differentiating Potentially Low from Average and High First Grade Readers," *Journal of Educational Research*, 53 (1960), 300–304.

168. Myklebust, Helmer. "Psychoneurological Learning Disorders in Children," in S. Kirk and W. Becker (eds.), *Conference on Children with Minimal Brain Impairment*. Chicago: Easter Seal Research Foundation, National Society for Crippled Children and Adults, 1963.

169. Myklebust, Helmer, and Boshes, Benjamin. "Psychoneurological Learning Disorders in Children," *Archives of Pediatrics*, 77 (1960), 247–256.

170. Natchez, Gladys. *Personality Patterns and Oral Reading*. New York: New York University Press, 1959.

171. Nicholson, Alice. "Background Abilities Related to Reading Success in First Grade," *Journal of Education*, 140 (1958), 7–24.

172. Novick, Jack. "Stress as Represented by Premature First-Grade Placement and Its Effect on the Psychological Development of Young Children," *American Journal of Orthopsychiatry*, 33 (1963), 332.

173. Olson, Willard C. *Child Development*. Boston: D. C. Heath & Co., 1959.

174. Oppé, Thomas. "Emotional Aspects of Prematurity," *Cerebral Palsy Bulletin*, 2 (1960), 233–237.

175. Orton, Samuel T. "Familial Occurrence of Disorders in Acquisition of Language," *Eugenics*, 3 (1930), 140–147.

176. ———. "Special Disability in Spelling," *Bulletin of the Neurological Institute in New York*, 1 (1931), 159–192.

177. ———. *Reading, Writing and Speech Problems in Children.* New York: Norton & Co., 1937.

178. Oseretzky, N. "Psychomotorik, Methoden zur Untersuchung der Motorik," [Beihefte zur] Supplement to *Zeitschrift fuer Angewandte Psychologie*, 57 (1931), 1–162.

179. Otto, Wayne. "Family Position and Success in Reading," *Reading Teacher*, 19 (1965), 119–123.

180. Pasamanick, Benjamin and Knobloch, Hilda. "Brain Damage and Reproductive Casualty," *American Journal of Orthopsychiatry*, 30 (1960), 298–305.

181. Pearson, Gerald H. J. "A Survey of Learning Difficulties in Children," *Psychoanalytic Study of the Child*, 7 (1952), 322–386.

182. ———. *Psychoanalysis and the Education of the Child.* New York: Norton & Co., 1954.

183. Pestalozzi, Johann. *Education of Man, Aphorisms.* New York: Philosophical Library, 1951.

184. Petty, Mary C. "An Experimental Study of Certain Factors Influencing Reading Readiness," *Journal of Educational Psychology*, 30 (1939), 215–230.

185. Piaget, Jean. *The Origins of Intelligence in Children.* New York: International Universities Press, 1952.

186. ———. *The Language and Thought of the Child.* New York: Humanities Press, 1959.

187. Plessas, Gus P. "Reading Abilities of High and Low Auders," *Elementary School Journal*, 63 (1963), 223–226.

188. Rabinovitch, Ralph. "Reading and Learning Disabilities," in S. Arieti (ed.), *American Handbook of Psychiatry.* Vol. I; New York: Basic Books, 1959.

189. Rabinovitch, Ralph, *et al.* "A Research Approach to Reading Retardation," *Association for Research in Nervous and Mental Disorders*, 34 (1954), 363–396.

190. Reed, Homer. "Some Relationships between Neurological Dys-

function and Behavioral Deficits in Children," in S. Kirk and W. Becker (eds.), *Conference on Children with Minimal Brain Impairment*. Chicago: Easter Seal Research Foundation, National Society of Crippled Children and Adults, 1963.

191. Regents' Conference on the Improvement of Reading. University of the State of New York, 1962.

192. Reynolds, Maynard Clinton. "A Study of the Relationships between Auditory Characteristics and Specific Silent Reading Abilities," *Journal of Educational Research*, 46 (1953), 439–449.

193. Riessman, Frank. *The Culturally Deprived Child*. New York: Harper & Row, 1962.

194. Robinson, Helen M. "Vision and Reading Difficulties. The Findings of Research on Visual Difficulties in Reading," in J. Allen Figurel (ed.), *Reading for Effective Living. Conference Proceedings of the International Reading Association*, 3 (1958), 107–111.

195. Rosen, Victor H. "Strephosymbolia: An Intrasystematic Disturbance of the Synthetic Function of the Ego," *Psychoanalytic Study of the Child*, 10 (1955), 83–99.

196. Ross, Alan D. "Integration as a Basic Central Function," *Psychological Reports Monograph*, Supplement 2 (1955).

197. Roswell, Florence, and Natchez, Gladys. *Reading Disability*. New York: Basic Books, 1964.

198. Rutherford, William. "Perceptual-Motor Training and Readiness," Paper presented at Tenth Annual Convention of the International Reading Association, Detroit, Mich., May 1965.

199. Sampson, Edward. "Birth Order, Need Achievement, and Conformity," *Journal of Abnormal and Social Psychology*, 64 (1962), 155–159.

200. Scarborough, Olive R., Hindsman, Edwin, and Hanna, Geneva. "Anxiety Level and Performance in School Subjects," *Psychological Reports*, 9 (1961), 425–430.

201. Schilder, Paul. *Contributions to Developmental Neuropsychiatry*. New York: International Universities Press, 1964.

202. Schuell, Hildred, Jenkins, James, and Jiménez-Pabón, Edward. *Aphasia in Adults*. New York: Harper & Row, 1964.

203. Sheldon, William D. "Language Skills of the Culturally Disadvantaged." Paper presented at Tenth Annual Convention of the International Reading Association, Detroit, Mich., May 1965.

204. Shire, Sister Mary Louise. "The Relation of Certain Linguistic Factors to Reading Achievement of First Grade Children." Ph.D. thesis, Fordham University, 1945.

205. Shirley, Hale F. "Etiology and Emotional Factors," *California Medicine*, 83 (1955), 81–84.

206. Silvaroli, Nicholas J. "Intellectual and Emotional Factors as Predictors of Children's Success in First Grade Reading." Paper presented at Tenth Annual Convention of the International Reading Association, Detroit, Mich., May 1965.

207. Silver, Archie A. "Diagnostic Value of Three Drawing Tests for Children," *Journal of Pediatrics*, 37 (1950), 120–143.

208. Silver, Archie A., and Hagin, Rosa. "Specific Reading Disability. Delineation of the Syndrome and Relationship to Cerebral Dominance," *Comprehensive Psychiatry*, 1 (1960), 126–134.

209. ———. "Specific Reading Disability. Follow-Up Studies," *American Journal of Orthopsychiatry*, 34 (1964), 95–102.

210. Silverman, William A. "The Outcome of Prematurity," in *Mental Retardation*. Proceedings of the Association for Research in Nervous and Mental Diseases. Baltimore: William and Wilkins, 1962.

211. Simon, Jean. "Une Batterie d'Épreuves Psychologiques pour la Prédiction de la Réussite en Lecture," *Enfance*, 5 (1952), 475–480.

212. ———. "Contribution à la Psychologie de la Lecture," *Enfance*, 7 (1954), 431–447.

213. Simon, Maria D. "Body Configuration and School Readiness," *Child Development*, 30 (1959), 493–512.

214. Slingerland, Beth H. "A Public School Program of Prevention for Young Children with Specific Language Disability," in *Dyslexia in Special Education* (Orton Society), Monograph I (1965).

215. Smith, Carol E., and Keogh, Barbara. "The Group Bender Gestalt Test as a Reading Readiness Screening Instrument," *Perceptual and Motor Skills*, 15 (1962), 639–645.

216. Smith, Nila B. "An Evaluation of Reading in American Schools," in J. Allen Figurel (ed.), *Challenge and Experiment in Reading. Conference Proceedings of the International Reading Association*, 7 (1962), 179–190.

217. Somers, Robert H. "A New Asymmetric Measure of Association

for Ordinal Variables," *American Sociological Review*, 27 (1962), 799–811.

218. Spencer, Ellen-Marie. "Investigation of the Maturation of Various Facets of Auditory Perception in Pre-School Children." Ph.D. thesis, Northwestern University, 1959.

219. Stamback, Mira. "Le Problème du Rhythme dans le Développement de l'Enfant et dans les Dyslexies d'Evolution," *Enfance*, 4 (1951), 480–502.

220. Strauss, Alfred A., and Lehtinen, Laura E. *Psychopathology and Education of Brain Injured Children*. New York: Grune & Stratton, 1947.

221. Strickland, Ruth. "The Language of Elementary School Children: Its Relationship to the Language of Reading Textbooks and the Quality of Reading of Selected Children," *Indiana University School of Education Bulletin*, 38 (1962), No. 4.

222. Subirana, Antonio. "The Problem of Cerebral Dominance: The Relationship Between Handedness and Language Function," *Logos*, 4 (1961), 67–85.

223. Swedish Royal Board of Education. *Laroplan for Grundskolan*. Stockholm, 1962.

224. Tanner, J. M. *Education and Physical Growth*. London: University of London Press, 1961.

225. Taylor, Earl A. "The Spans: Perception, Apprehension and Recognition," *American Journal of Ophthalmology*, 44 (1957), 501–507.

226. Teicher, Joseph. "Preliminary Survey of Motility in Children," *Quarterly Journal of Child Behavior*, 3 (1951), 460–491.

227. Templin, Mildred C. *Certain Language Skills in Children*. Minneapolis: University of Minnesota Press, 1957.

228. Thelander, H. E., Phelps, Jane K., and Kirk, E. Walton. "Learning Disabilities Associated with Lesser Brain Damage," *Journal of Pediatrics*, 53 (1958), 405–409.

229. Thomas, Alexander, *et al. Behavioral Individuality in Early Childhood*. New York: New York University Press, 1963.

230. Thompson, Bertha B. "A Longitudinal Study of Auditory Discrimination," *Journal of Educational Research*, 56 (1963), 376–378.

231. Tinker, Miles. "Eye Movements in Reading," *Journal of Educational Research*, 30 (1936), 241–277.

232. Uddenberg, Gunborg. "Diagnostic Studies in Prematures," *Acta Psychiatrica et Neurologica Scandinavica*, Supplement 104 (1955).

233. U.S. Bureau of the Census, *County and City Data, 1962* (A Statistical Abstract Supplement). Washington 25, D.C.: U.S. Government Printing Office, 1962, p. 536.

234. Van Hoosan, Marie. "Just Enough English," *Reading Teacher*, 18 (1965), 507.

235. Vernon, Magdalen D. *Backwardness in Reading. A Study of Its Nature and Origin*. New York: Cambridge University Press, 1958.

236. Vygotsky, Lev. *Thought and Language*. Cambridge, Mass.: MIT Press, 1962.

237. Washburne, Carleton. "Individualized Plan of Instruction in Winnetka—Adjusting Reading Programs to Individuals," *Supplementary Educational Monograph*, 52. Chicago: University of Chicago Press, 1941, pp. 90–95.

238. Wattenberg, William W., and Clifford, Clare. "Relation of Self-Concepts to Beginning Achievement in Reading," *Child Development*, 35 (1964), 461–467.

239. Weaver, Carl H., Furbee, Catherine, and Everhart, Rodney W. "Articulatory Competency and Reading Readiness," *Journal of Speech and Hearing Research*, 3 (1960), 174–180.

240. Weiner, Max, and Feldmann, Shirley. "Validation Studies of a Reading Prognosis Test for Children of Lower and Middle Socio-Economic Status," *Educational and Psychological Measurement*, 23 (1963), 807–814.

241. Weiss, Deso. *Cluttering*. Foundations of Speech Pathology Series. Englewood Cliffs, N.J.: Prentice-Hall, Inc., 1964.

242. Wenar, Charles. "The Reliability of Mothers' Histories," *Child Development*, 32 (1961), 491–500.

243. Wepman, Joseph. *Auditory Discrimination Test*. Chicago: Language Research Associates, 1958.

244. ———. "Auditory Discrimination, Speech, and Reading," *Elementary School Journal*, 60 (1960), 325–333.

245. ———. "Interrelationship of Hearing, Speech and Reading," *Reading Teacher*, 14 (1961), 245–247.

246. Werner, Heinz. "The Concept of Development from a Comparative and Organismic Point of View," in D. B. Harris (ed.), *The*

Concept of Development. Minneapolis: University of Minnesota Press, 1957.

247. Werner, Heinz, and Kaplan, Bernard. *Symbol Formation.* New York: Wiley, 1963.

248. White, Robert W. "Ego Reality in Psychoanalytic Terms," *Psychological Issues,* 3 (1963), No. 3.

249. Wiener, Gerald. "Psychologic Correlates of Premature Birth: A Review," *Journal of Nervous and Mental Diseases,* 134 (1962), 129–144.

250. Wiener, Gerald, *et al.* "Correlates of Low Birth Weight: Psychological Status at Six to Seven Years of Age," *Pediatrics,* 35 (1965), 434–444.

251. Wood, Nancy E. *Language Development and Language Disorders: A Compendium of Lectures.* Monograph of the Society for Research in Child Development, Purdue University, Serial No. 77, 25 (1960).

252. Wortis, Helen, and Freedman, Alfred M. "The Contribution of Social Environment to the Development of Premature Children," *American Journal of Orthopsychiatry,* 35 (1965), 57–68.

253. Yedinack, Jeanette. "A Study of the Linguistic Functioning of Children with Articulation and Reading Disabilities," *Journal of Genetic Psychology,* 74 (1949), 23–59.

254. Zangwill, Oliver L. "Dyslexia in Relation to Cerebral Dominance," in J. Money (ed.), *Reading Disability, Progress and Research Needs in Dyslexia.* Baltimore: Johns Hopkins Press, 1962.

255. Zaporozhets, Alexander V. "The Development of Perception in the Preschool Child," *Child Development Monographs,* Serial No. 100, 30 (1965), No. 2.

Sources

◆

AJURIAGUERRA, JULIAN DE. "Les Troubles du Langage," *Confinia Neurologica*, 23 (1963), 91–107.

AUSTIN, MARY C., and MORRISON, COLEMAN. *The First R: The Harvard Report on Reading in Elementary Schools*. New York: Macmillan, 1963.

BENDER, LAURETTA. "Problems in Conceptualization and Communication in Children with Developmental Alexia," in P. HOCH and J. ZUBIN (eds.), *Psychopathology of Communication*. New York: Grune & Stratton, 1958.

———. *Psychopathology of Children with Organic Brain Disorders*. Springfield, Ill.: Chas. C. Thomas, 1956.

BIRCH, HERBERT G. "The Problem of 'Brain Damage' in Children," in H. BIRCH (ed.), *Brain Damage in Children*. Baltimore: Williams and Wilkins, 1964.

BOREL-MAISONNY, SUZANNE. "Les Troubles du Langage dans les Dyslexies et les Dysorthographies," *Enfance*, 4 (1951), 400–444.

BRYANT, N. DALE. "Reading Disability: Part of a Syndrome of Neurological Dysfunctioning," in J. ALLEN FIGUREL (ed.), *Challenge and Experiment in Reading. Conference Proceedings of the International Reading Association*, 7 (1962), 139–143.

CRITCHLEY, MACDONALD. *Developmental Dyslexia*. London: Wm. Heinemann Medical Books, 1964.

CRUICKSHANK, WILLIAM, *et al*. *A Teaching Method for Brain-Injured and Hyperactive Children*. Syracuse: Syracuse University Press, 1961.

DEUTSCH, CYNTHIA. "Physiological and Perceptual Factors in Reading." Paper read at Tenth Annual Convention of the International Reading Association, Detroit, Mich., May 1965.

DEUTSCH, MARTIN. "The Role of Social Class in Language Development and Cognition," *American Journal of Orthopsychiatry*, 35 (1965), 78–88.

DRILLIEN, CECIL. *The Growth and Development of the Prematurely Born Infant.* Baltimore: Williams & Wilkins, 1964.

DURRELL, DONALD. *Improving Reading Instruction.* Tarrytown, N.Y.: World Books, 1956.

ESCALONA, SIBYLLE, and HEIDER, GRACE. *Prediction and Outcome.* New York: Basic Books, 1959.

FREEDMAN, ALFRED M., *et al.* "The Influence of Hyperbilirubinaemia on the Early Development of the Premature," *Psychiatric Research Report, American Psychiatric Association*, 13 (1960), 108–127.

GALLAGHER, J. ROSWELL. "Specific Language Disability (Dyslexia)," *Clinical Proceedings, Children's Hospital, Washington, D.C.*, 16 (1960), 3–15.

GATES, ARTHUR, and BOND, GUY. "Factors Determining Success and Failure in Beginning Reading," in C. W. HUNNICUTT and W. J. IVERSON (eds.), *Research in the Three R's.* New York: Harper & Row, 1958.

GESELL, ARNOLD. *The Embryology of Behavior—The Beginning of the Human Mind.* New York: Harper & Row, 1945.

GESELL, ARNOLD, and ILG, FRANCES. *The Child from Five to Ten.* New York: Harper & Row, 1946.

HALLGREN, BERTIL. "Specific Dyslexia: A Clinical and Genetic Study," *Acta Psychiatrica et Neurologica*, Supplement 65 (1950).

———. "Perceptual Difficulties in Reading Disability." Paper read at Pre-Conference Institute of the Annual Meeting of the International Reading Association, May 1961.

HEBB, DONALD. *Organization of Behavior.* New York: Wiley, 1949.

HERMANN, KNUD. *Reading Disability: A Medical Study of Word-Blindness and Related Handicaps.* Springfield, Ill.: Chas. C. Thomas, 1959.

DE HIRSCH, KATRINA. "Specific Dyslexia or Strephosymbolia," *Folia Phoniatrica*, 4 (1952), 231–248.

———. "Tests Designed to Discover Potential Reading Difficulties at the Six-Year-Old Level," *American Journal of Orthopsychiatry*, 27 (1957), 566–576.

————. "Concepts Related to Normal Reading Processes and Their Application to Reading Pathology," *Journal of Genetic Psychology*, 102 (1963), 277–285.

ILG, FRANCES, and AMES, LOUISE. *School Readiness*. New York: Harper & Row, 1964.

JANSKY, JEANNETTE. "A Case of Severe Dyslexia with Aphasic-Like Symptoms," *Reading Teacher*, 15 (1961), 110–113.

KEPHART, NEWELL. *The Slow Learner in the Classroom*. Columbus, Ohio: Charles E. Merrill Books, 1960.

LANGMAN, MURIEL POTTER. "The Reading Process: A Descriptive Interdisciplinary Approach," *Genetic Psychology Monographs*, 62 (1960).

LASHLEY, KARL. "The Problem of Serial Order in Behavior," in L. A. JEFFRESS (ed.), *Cerebral Mechanisms in Behavior*. New York: Wiley, 1954.

MALMQUIST, EVE. *Factors Related to Reading Disabilities in the First Grade of the Elementary School*. Stockholm: Almquist & Wiksell, 1958.

MASLAND, MARY W., and CASE, LINDA. "Limitation of Auditory Memory as a Factor in Delayed Language Development." Paper read at Meeting of the International Association for Logopedics and Phoniatrics, Vienna, August 1965.

MASLAND, RICHARD. "The Neurologic Substrata of Communicative Disorders." Paper read at the Annual Meeting of the American Speech and Hearing Association, Chicago, November 1965.

McCARTHY, DOROTHEA. "The Language Development of the Preschool Child," *University of Minnesota Child Welfare Monograph*, 4 (1930).

MONROE, MARION. *Children Who Cannot Read*. Chicago: Chicago University Press, 1932.

MYKLEBUST, HELMER, and JOHNSON, DORIS. "Dyslexia in Children," *Exceptional Children*, 29 (1962), 14–25.

ORTON, SAMUEL. *Reading, Writing and Speech Problems in Children*. New York: Norton & Co., 1937.

PEARSON, GERALD H. J. *Psychoanalysis and the Education of the Child*. New York: Norton & Co., 1954.

PIAGET, JEAN. *The Language and Thought of the Child*. New York: Humanities Press, 1959.

RABINOVITCH, RALPH, et al. "A Research Approach to Reading Retardation," *Association for Research in Nervous and Mental Disorders*, 34 (1954), 363–396.

SCHILDER, PAUL. *Contributions to Developmental Neuropsychiatry.* New York: International University Press, 1964.

SHANKWEILER, DONALD. "Developmental Dyslexia," *Cortex*, 1 (1964), 54–62.

SILVER, ARCHIE, and HAGIN, ROSA. "Maturation of Perceptual Functions in Children with Specific Reading Disability," *Reading Teacher*, 19 (1966), 253–259.

SILVERMAN, WILLIAM A. *Dunham's Premature Infants.* 3rd ed.; New York: Harper & Row, 1961.

STRAUSS, ALFRED, and LEHTINEN, LAURA. *Psychopathology and Education of the Brain-Injured Child.* New York: Grune & Stratton, 1947.

SUBIRANA, ANTONIO. "The Problem of Cerebral Dominance: The Relationship between Handedness and Language Function," *Logos*, 4 (1961), 67–85.

TANNER, J. M. *Education and Physical Growth.* London: University of London Press, 1961.

TEMPLIN, MILDRED. *Certain Language Skills in Children.* Minneapolis: University of Minnesota Press, 1957.

VERNON, MAGDALEN D. *Backwardness in Reading. A Study of Its Nature and Origin.* New York: Cambridge University Press, 1958.

VYGOTSKY, LEV. *Thought and Language.* Cambridge, Mass.: MIT Press, 1962.

WERNER, HEINZ. "The Concept of Development from a Comparative and Organismic Point of View," in D. B. HARRIS (ed.), *The Concept of Development.* Minneapolis: University of Minnesota Press, 1957.

WIENER, GERALD, et al. "Correlates of Low Birth Weight: Psychological Status at Six to Seven Years of Age," *Pediatrics*, 35 (1965), 434–444.

WOOD, NANCY. *Language Development and Language Disorders: A Compendium of Lectures.* Monograph of the Society for Research in Child Development, Purdue University, Serial No. 77, 25 (1960).

ZANGWILL, OLIVER L. *Cerebral Dominance and Its Relation to Psychological Function.* London: Oliver & Boyd, 1960.

Terms

*Technical terms not found here are defined operationally in
the text and can be found in the index.*

AFFECT—A feeling state.

AUDING—The perceiving, processing, storing, and recalling of auditory
verbal sequences.

CHI SQUARE—A means of estimating whether a given distribution
differs from expected values to such a degree as to show evidence
for the operation of non-chance factors.

DEFICIT—If used in combination with "neurological" and "language"
it means impairment of functioning which may or may not be due
to structural change.

DYSFUNCTION—Disordered functioning.

HYPERKINETIC—Hyperactive.

LIBIDINAL CATHEXIS—The libido or psychic energy that has been in-
vested in an object, person, etc.

ORGANISMIC—Pertaining to functioning of the total organism.

PATHOGNOMONIC—Characteristic of a disease or disorder.

PROPRIOCEPTIVE—Referring to sensations arising from muscles, ten-
dons, joints.

SEQUELAE—Any affection following and caused by a previous disease.

TAU BETA (tau coefficient of correlation)—A rank order correlation
(where the score is based on the comparison of the rank of each
item compared with each other item).

d_{yx} Like tau beta, a rank order correlation that is not dependent on
normal distribution of data.

p Probability that a given event might occur by chance.

INDEX